The
Tinnitus
Retraining Therapy
Book

The Tinnitus Retraining Therapy Book

WALKING YOU THROUGH TRT

James A. Henry

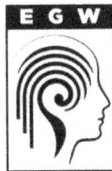

Ears Gone Wrong, LLC

ISBN: 978-1-962629-01-0 (paperback)
ISBN: 978-1-962629-02-7 (ebook)
ISBN: 978-1-962629-00-3 (hardcover)

Contents

Foreword

I love this book!

The author is knowledgeable, experienced, and dedicated. He is a man of consummate integrity, universally respected in both the clinical and research tinnitus communities. To those who know him and his work, Jim Henry is truly a tinnitus superstar.

In *The Tinnitus Retraining Therapy Book: Walking You Through TRT*, Dr. Henry takes you by the hand as together you navigate the challenging waters of TRT. Here you have one of the world's leading authorities chatting with you instead of preaching at you. Refreshing, no?

When I was a TRT patient back in the mid-1990s, things were rather simple. There was only one TRT clinician in the US, and you knew that you were getting the real thing because it was that TRT clinician, Dr. Pawel Jastreboff, who conceived the model and developed the protocols. The difficulty today stems from the fact that with TRT there is no standardization. Since the name "Tinnitus Retraining Therapy" has never been copyrighted, anybody can do just about anything and call it TRT. Further complicating matters is the fact that with TRT there is no certification. Even if a licensed health care provider has taken a formal TRT course, you have no assurance that he or she has understood the material and is applying it correctly. Then there is the internet, where you can find seemingly limitless well-intended posts about TRT. The problem is that just because a post might make good sense, that does not mean it contains good information. And most of the internet posts about TRT contain horrible information.

This book contains good information. This book contains great information. This book is important. This book is necessary. I do love this book!

Stephen M. Nagler, MD
Atlanta, Georgia

Preface

I spent the great majority of my professional career studying tinnitus. More specifically, I studied methods of tinnitus evaluation and treatment that would be used in a clinical setting. I have always been concerned about the lack of standards for tinnitus clinical services, and one of my overall objectives was to provide evidence for how to conduct a tinnitus clinical assessment and perform effective treatment for bothersome tinnitus.

Early in my career I kept hearing about Tinnitus Retraining Therapy (TRT), which was getting a lot of attention in the 1990s. Dr. Pawel Jastreboff was the developer of TRT, and it was first used in a clinic in London in 1988 by Mr. Jonathan W.P. Hazell, an otolaryngologist, along with his audiologist Jacqueline Sheldrake. Dr. Jastreboff published a pivotal article in 1990 that laid out the basic idea for his *neurophysiological model*, which underlies everything that is done with TRT.

Neurophysiological model—hang in there with me. Neurophysiological is a big word that may be unfamiliar to you. *Neuro* refers to nerves, and *physiological* refers to how the nerves function (in the brain, with respect to tinnitus). The neurophysiological model shows how different parts of the brain are involved when a person has tinnitus. Some of those parts need to be "disconnected" when tinnitus causes stress and emotional reactions. The TRT counseling explains all of this in detail.

Dr. Jastreboff started giving multiday training seminars to teach clinicians how to conduct TRT. I attended one of his first seminars in 1997, which was an eye-opener for me in many ways. I learned new concepts about tinnitus and became motivated to conduct a controlled research study to evaluate the effectiveness of TRT. I wrote a grant proposal for this purpose and received funding to perform the study over four years. I personally provided the TRT counseling to 64 participants in the study. Each participant required five counseling sessions over an 18-month period. On average, they improved progressively over the period of treatment.

TRT counseling—what exactly does that refer to? *Counseling* is a word that is frequently used by audiologists in general practice as well as TRT clinicians. It is also widely used by psychologists. TRT counseling should not be thought of as psychotherapy. It is more of a back-and-forth educational process between the clinician and the recipient of the counseling.

I received funding for another study to provide TRT counseling to groups of people. I personally delivered the counseling for that study as well. *Group TRT counseling* also got good results, but not as good as the individualized counseling in my first study. I ended up writing many articles about TRT and gave related presentations and training seminars. I also wrote two books about TRT that were directed to professionals. The present book is directed to the general public.

Probably the greatest challenge to anyone who desires treatment with TRT is finding a practitioner who fully grasps and can accurately deliver the structured counseling. The counseling is, without question, quite detailed and difficult for many people to understand. This book attempts to address that concern by providing word-for-word counseling directly to you, the reader.

Prior to receiving the counseling, you will be evaluated for TRT using the recommended test procedures. Most importantly, you will respond to the questions from the TRT Initial Interview. This in-depth interview is designed to get at the root of your tinnitus problem and also to assess for any sound tolerance or hearing problems. Your responses provide critical information to determine which of five treatment categories would be most appropriate for you.

The overall intent of this book is to provide detailed information about TRT to anyone who might be interested—no prior knowledge necessary (although you may be interested in reading my previous book, *The Tinnitus Book: Understanding Tinnitus and How to Find Relief*, for more general information about tinnitus). The level of detail about TRT in the present book has not previously been made available to the general public. Detailed descriptions of TRT have been available to clinicians and researchers for years, but those books are relatively expensive and contain technical language that would be difficult for the average person to comprehend.

This book supplements the original TRT book (by Jastreboff and Hazell), the TRT instructional courses, and the many previous articles, books, and book chapters about TRT. What sets this book apart is the detailed reader-oriented clinical procedures that are described, as well as the unique perspectives on the neurophysiological model and other aspects of the TRT program. It is all intended to educate you as to what Jastreboff and Hazell described in their 2004 book, which is the definitive resource for TRT. My efforts have gone into making this information available and accessible to the average person. In spite of my attempts to simplify and clarify everything, it's a lot to learn. My suggestion is to read through the information slowly and carefully. Take your time and try to understand each topic. I truly hope this book is of great value to you!

Note to the Reader

This book is intended to provide educational information about tinnitus and related auditory problems. It cannot be construed as providing any form of therapy or treatment. If you have any of the symptoms described in this book and feel that professional services are needed, you need to meet with an appropriate healthcare provider.

PART 1

Introduction and Background

CHAPTER 1

Abigail and Robert

Abigail is a 52-year-old server at a local steak house restaurant. She has been serving food and drinks all her life, and she worked in bars during her younger years. She described the bars as "extremely noisy with blaring music." To communicate with customers, they often had to "yell in each other's ears." After doing this kind of work for over 10 years, she decided she would rather work in a (relatively) quiet restaurant.

One day, while working in the restaurant, another server dropped a tray of dishes right next to Abigail. The sound of the crashing dishes startled her and "sounded like an explosion." She immediately noticed that her ears started ringing. While she was lying in bed that night, the ringing was still there. To her surprise, and dismay, the ringing persisted over the next few weeks.

Abigail began to worry that her ears were seriously damaged and became fixated on listening to her tinnitus, which caused a great deal of distress. She made an appointment with an ear, nose, and throat (ENT) physician, hoping some kind of cure would be available. The doctor told her "nothing could be done about it" and prescribed anti-anxiety medication. Abigail started taking the medication on a regular basis, which "took the edge off the stress caused by the tinnitus." Over time, however, the medication was not helpful—she continued to think about, and react to, her tinnitus.

She gradually weaned herself off the medication and began a serious internet search for anything that might help her. She was overwhelmed with the number of websites that appeared. Some were for different clinics that specialized in tinnitus treatment, while others promoted books, devices, and remote (online) treatment. Many more offered various pills, with some even claiming to cure tinnitus. A cure—complete elimination of her tinnitus—is what she was looking for. She purchased a bottle of pills that had a catchy name relating to stopping tinnitus. She took the pills for a month with no effect. She then tried a different brand of pills, but they too were ineffective.

Feeling discouraged, she decided to make an appointment at a clinic that advertised tinnitus services. She visited with an audiologist there who said he was trained in Tinnitus Retraining Therapy (TRT). He conducted a full evaluation and said that Abigail was a TRT "category 2" patient. That meant she had bothersome tinnitus along with significant hearing difficulties. She was aware of the tinnitus but hadn't realized she also had hearing loss. She had thought that her hearing difficulties were due to her tinnitus.

Part of the treatment was wearing hearing aids that had a built-in sound generator (that emitted a "shhh"-type sound). She used the hearing aids for a few weeks and then came back to the clinic for her first TRT counseling appointment. The audiologist adjusted her hearing aids and also activated the sound generator in each one. The volume of the sound generators was adjusted to be "close to but below the mixing point," which the audiologist explained was a tiny bit below the volume level at which the noise from the sound generator and the tinnitus just begin to mix or blend together.

The counseling was extensive and required two sessions to cover all of the material. The counseling was based on the TRT neurophysiological model, which explains what goes on in the brain when tinnitus is bothersome. The information made sense to Abigail, and she wore the hearing aids and attended additional appointments over the next year. The objective of the treatment was to facilitate *habituation*—to stop reacting to the tinnitus and to not be aware of it most of the time. She was skeptical that this goal could be achieved but noticed after six months that habituation seemed to have started. After one year, she felt that she had almost fully habituated to her tinnitus and that no further treatment was needed.

> The objective of the treatment was to facilitate *habituation*—to stop reacting to the tinnitus and to not be aware of it most of the time.

Robert

Robert is a physician who works in a pathology lab at a university hospital. Most of his time at work is spent looking at tissue samples through a microscope to determine whether cancer is present. His work environment is very quiet, and he has never been exposed to significant amounts of loud noise. He in fact prefers quiet and has always avoided noisy settings.

He woke up one morning and noticed a high-pitched "whining" sound in his ears. He at first didn't think much of it, but over the next few days became concerned because the sound did not quit. He contacted an audiologist who worked at his hospital, and the audiologist evaluated his hearing. Robert had normal hearing sensitivity and so hearing aids were not recommended. The audiologist answered some questions Robert had about his tinnitus but was unable to provide further help other than to recommend that Robert meet with a psychologist.

Robert made an appointment with a psychologist to discuss his tinnitus problem. The psychologist knew very little about tinnitus but did the best she could to counsel Robert to basically try to ignore it. After a few meetings, Robert became frustrated with the lack of progress and decided not to continue the sessions.

Just like Abigail (described above), Robert started searching the internet to find out what he could do about his tinnitus. He was not interested in taking any pills and searched for a tinnitus specialist who was fairly close to home. He found one who specialized in TRT and made an appointment. The audiologist confirmed that Robert had normal hearing along with his bothersome tinnitus, which meant Robert was a TRT "category 1" patient.

Robert agreed to participate in receiving TRT. He was fit with ear-level sound generators, and the audiologist explained how to adjust the sound to "close to but below the mixing point." Robert attended the TRT counseling sessions with the audiologist, where he learned about the neurophysiological model and how habituation could be achieved.

Robert never did learn why he had a sudden onset of tinnitus, but he suspected it was due to a combination of stressors in his life, in both his job and his personal relationships. Wearing the sound generators did not seem to help at first, but the audiologist explained the purpose of the sound generators and recommended that he *avoid silence*. Robert didn't want to give up his silence, but he agreed to enrich his sound environment with low-level sound both at work and at home. Being a physician, he fully understood the neurophysiological model, how it explained why his tinnitus was so bothersome, and why the TRT treatment should be effective in promoting habituation. The treatment was indeed effective. At one point, Robert realized that even in quiet situations he wasn't thinking about his tinnitus. Basically, he was just fine—even in silence. Simply put, his "new normal" was not to care (or be concerned) about his tinnitus. It became a non-issue in his life.

> At one point, Robert realized that even in quiet situations he wasn't thinking about his tinnitus.

Where Do We Go from Here?

Abigail and Robert were both fortunate that they found good help for their tinnitus problems. That is not always the outcome for people who are distressed by tinnitus. Finding a qualified tinnitus specialist can be challenging because there are no official standards for the clinical management of tinnitus. This lack of standards is unfortunately the situation everywhere in the world.[1,2]

> Finding a qualified tinnitus specialist can be challenging because there are no official standards for the clinical management of tinnitus.

This book focuses on one form of tinnitus management: Tinnitus Retraining Therapy (TRT)—the method received by Abigail and Robert. TRT is one of a handful of clinical treatments I would recommend to anyone who needs help for bothersome tinnitus.[3]

We're of course back to the same concern that finding a TRT provider can be difficult. And finding a *competent* TRT provider can be even more difficult. Any clinician can hang out a shingle and claim to be a tinnitus expert. They can also hang out a shingle and claim to be a TRT expert. After reading this book, you will be in a better position to evaluate any claims of TRT expertise.

Formal TRT training has been made available by the founder of TRT (Dr. Pawel Jastreboff) since the mid-1990s. TRT providers should have completed that training. Just completing the training, however, does not ensure that TRT will be conducted in the proper manner. TRT can be difficult to learn—it needs to be fully understood in order to properly implement the procedures.[4]

If you are considering TRT, make sure your provider has received the formal training. Ask the provider when the training was received, who delivered the training, how many patients the provider has treated with TRT, and how successful the treatment has been. You need to be satisfied that your provider has been properly trained and is experienced and competent in delivering TRT successfully to many patients.

You might be wondering, "What is the evidence that TRT works?" If so, that's the right question to ask. For full transparency, you should be aware of what the scientific literature says about treatment with TRT. This is a fairly tedious topic to cover, so I've moved that section to appendix A for those who are interested.

> ...you should be aware of what the scientific literature says about treatment with TRT.

Suggestions for Getting the Most Benefit from This Book

It is likely that you, the reader, have tinnitus yourself, or you have a family member or friend who has tinnitus. Or maybe you're a clinician who wants to learn more about TRT. If you've searched the internet to learn about tinnitus and/or TRT, you may be confused due to all the conflicting information about tinnitus that is found there. Lack of standards is the problem.

My first book in this Ears Gone Wrong series, *The Tinnitus Book: Understanding Tinnitus and How to Find Relief,* provides a thorough description of tinnitus, how and why it affects people, and what can be done about it.[3] The present book focuses specifically on TRT, which is one of the few methods I am comfortable recommending—the others being cognitive behavioral therapy (CBT and *third wave* CBT), Progressive Tinnitus Management (PTM) and its telehealth version (Tele-PTM), and Tinnitus Activities Treatment (TAT). My first book provides a summary of each of these methods.

While much of TRT can be very technical, I've attempted to describe it in a way that would be understandable to anyone. The next four chapters (2, 3, 4, and 5) focus on how people with tinnitus would receive a clinical evaluation for their tinnitus, which would determine their placement into one of five possible treatment categories.

Starting with chapter 4, I will be your TRT practitioner speaking directly to you, the patient. In chapter 5, I will walk you through the questions from the TRT Initial Interview. These questions are critical to diagnose your condition and to place you in the proper treatment category. In chapters 6, 7, and 8, I will walk you through your treatment sessions. Chapter 6 is an explanation of TRT sound therapy. Chapter 7 is background information to help

> Starting with chapter 4, I will be your TRT practitioner speaking directly to you, the patient.

understand the TRT neurophysiological model. Chapter 8 is an explanation of the neurophysiological model. In chapter 9, I will walk you through your six-month follow-up visit. Chapter 10 is a summary and wrap-up of the various concepts, along with TRT resources and tips for how to receive optimum benefit from TRT.

TRT was first used clinically in 1988,[5] and its use has since expanded around the world. It is a well-established method that is often misunderstood. This book can be useful to anyone who wishes to learn the details of TRT. The book is *not* intended to take the place of a competent TRT provider. The best way to receive TRT is directly from a provider who can skillfully lead you down the path toward habituation of every aspect of your tinnitus.

The Big Picture

I want to make sure you have realistic expectations about TRT and about methods of tinnitus management in general. As I already mentioned, a detailed description of tinnitus and how and why it affects people is included in my first book of this Ears Gone Wrong series.[3] I therefore will not repeat that information here. That information is *not* critical for you to benefit from this book, which is designed to get right at how you would be evaluated and treated with TRT.

A few comments are necessary to set the stage for the remainder of the book. When we refer to tinnitus, we are referring to the sensation of *sound* that is produced and perceived inside your head. It is important to separate that sound from any effects *caused by* the sound. Eliminating the sound would be a cure, and no one has yet discovered a cure for tinnitus—in spite of all the claims found on the internet. Treatment, therefore, has the goal of reducing or eliminating any *effects* caused by tinnitus. Those effects relate mainly to disrupted sleep, difficulty concentrating, and emotional reactions. Whether it's TRT or any other form of treatment, reducing or eliminating the effects of tinnitus is the realistic goal.

> Whether it's TRT or any other form of treatment, reducing or eliminating the effects of tinnitus is the realistic goal.

My advice to anyone is, first and foremost, become informed about tinnitus and how it can be managed. Becoming so informed is not necessarily easy due to the proliferation of false and misleading information on the internet and elsewhere. People with tinnitus may be desperate for help, and there is no end of fraudsters trying to take advantage of desperate people. The products and services that are offered may seem believable because of clever and persuasive marketing techniques that usually involve some partial truths. Becoming well informed is the best defense to avoid being coerced into purchasing unnecessary, ineffective, or worthless remedies.

The methods I am comfortable recommending (TRT, CBT and third wave CBT, PTM and Tele-PTM, and TAT) have all been around for many years. My belief is that clinicians who are proficient in any of these methods will get overall good results with their patients. No one method of treatment for tinnitus has been proven to be more effective than any other.

Because this is a book about TRT, that is where the focus will remain. In my previous book I described the different methods I am comfortable recommending along with resources to obtain more information about each.[3] A rudimentary knowledge about how these methods are alike and how they differ will be helpful in your quest to find quality tinnitus services. If you are unable to successfully help yourself with the available resources, it is essential to find an experienced, qualified provider who prioritizes the best interests of patients above any fees or profit. If a list of such providers were available, I certainly would share it with you. It unfortunately is not, which is due to the lack of standardization and regulation of tinnitus clinical services.

My hope is that this book will help to offset any difficulty in finding a competent tinnitus specialist. Whether it's TRT or any of the other well-established methods, such clinicians are in short supply. The content of this book is written in such a way as to optimize the potential for you, the reader, to learn the principles of TRT. I have made every effort to make this information accessible and practical. Information is power, and the information contained in this book will empower you whenever you are communicating with a provider who claims to specialize in tinnitus services.

PART 2

Evaluation for TRT

CHAPTER 2

Overview of TRT Evaluation Procedures

Clinical evaluation for TRT has been explained in numerous publications by the founders of TRT.[5-8] It has also been described in publications I have authored.[9-11] Perhaps the most definitive source to know exactly what evaluation procedures are recommended is chapter 3 in the book by Jastreboff and Hazell (2004).[4]

In this chapter we will discuss an overview of the evaluation procedures. In chapter 3, I will describe how patients are categorized to determine which variation of treatment would be most appropriate, and I will provide examples of patients in each of the five categories. In chapters 4 and 5, I will walk you through your evaluation appointment with a TRT practitioner. I will be the practitioner speaking directly to you, the patient, and describing your responses, which will be typical of many patients who undergo TRT. It will also be an education session to explain why you are asked each question and to provide general information about tinnitus that should be helpful to you.

Purpose of the Evaluation

The overall purpose of the evaluation is to diagnose and distinguish between concerns relating to hearing loss, tinnitus, and decreased sound tolerance.[7] In other words, how much of a problem is each of these three potential auditory conditions? The procedures include a physical examination, medical history, history of hearing loss, tinnitus, and decreased sound tolerance (using the TRT Initial Interview), a tinnitus questionnaire, and a hearing evaluation by an audiologist (audiological assessment).[4]

> The overall purpose of the evaluation is to diagnose and distinguish between concerns relating to hearing loss, tinnitus, and decreased sound tolerance.

Physical Examination

The physical examination is an important part of the TRT protocol and should be completed prior to the evaluation visit.[4] A physical exam is also recommended by all clinical practice guidelines for tinnitus that have been published to date.[12,13] The examination should be conducted by an ear-specialist physician such as an otolaryngologist, otologist, or neurotologist. The exam's purpose is "to detect any medical problems which may cause, contribute to, or have an impact on the treatment of tinnitus. This is essential in creating the basis for assurance that there is nothing medically wrong, requiring separate treatment, that can be linked to tinnitus or decreased sound tolerance."[4] (p. 76)

Medical History

Ideally, the medical history form is mailed out to patients and returned prior to the initial visit. This information is reviewed by the examiner before meeting with the patient. Otherwise, the medical history can be conducted in person at the beginning of the visit. The medical history is necessary to find out if there are any symptoms or conditions that would indicate the need for special services or referral to a different specialty.

There is no standardized set of questions for a medical history. The American Academy of Otolaryngology–Head and Neck Surgery Foundation (AAO-HNSF), however, has provided a list of key signs and symptoms that "dictate the need for referral" to a different specialty.[14] Appendix B reviews in some detail the AAO-HNSF recommendations for performing a medical history with patients who have tinnitus.

TRT Initial Interview

An initial in-person interview is conducted with each patient. A structured interview form is available for this purpose.[4,11]

Many excellent TRT clinicians, however, do not use a structured interview form. They know the areas to cover in the initial interview, and they do so in an unstructured manner. For the initial visit with you, the reader, we will use the structured interview form. "Taking a proper history, using TRT interview forms, is essential in selecting the correct treatment category.... The initial interview helps to evaluate the patient's problem and the degree of distress caused by it."[4] (p. 66) The TRT Initial Interview is described in detail in chapter 5.

> For the initial visit with you, the reader, we will use the structured interview form.

Hearing Evaluation

The hearing evaluation involves a number of tests conducted by an audiologist. Some of these tests are considered essential while others are not. Essential audiological tests include a basic hearing test (pure-tone audiometry) to obtain an audiogram, speech discrimination testing (to evaluate the ability to distinguish between different spoken words), and loudness discomfort level testing to evaluate for a loudness tolerance problem (hyperacusis). The full battery of audiological tests used for TRT is described in appendix C.

Tinnitus Questionnaire

A tinnitus questionnaire supplements the information that is obtained with the TRT Initial Interview. Individual questions in the Initial Interview provide numbers that quantify certain problem areas. A tinnitus questionnaire provides a single number that quantifies the overall tinnitus condition. Having such a number before, during, and after treatment is useful for evaluating the overall effectiveness of the treatment.

Dr. Jastreboff wrote, "While information provided by [the TRT Initial Interview] gives good insight into many aspects of tinnitus including its severity, the Tinnitus Handicap Inventory (THI) is used as well to assess tinnitus severity in a more formal manner."[5] (p. 585) The THI is a well-established tinnitus questionnaire that has been used in many TRT trials and in clinics that provide TRT.

In addition to the THI, many other questionnaires are available to assess how much a person's life is impacted by tinnitus.[14-16] All tinnitus questionnaires provide a total (index) score that typically ranges from 0 (no impact due to tinnitus) to 100 (maximum impact due to tinnitus).

Tinnitus questionnaires are also used to determine the *effectiveness* of treatment. A reduction in the index score (compared to the pre-treatment score) indicates improvement. Using a questionnaire for this purpose depends on the questionnaire's *responsiveness*, meaning the questionnaire's *sensitivity to detect change* in a person's tinnitus condition (better, worse, or no change). The Tinnitus

Functional Index (TFI) was the first tinnitus questionnaire to be validated for responsiveness.[17]

Developing the TFI required four years of effort and multiple stages of development using over 300 patients in each of stages 1 and 2.[17,18] The TFI has 25 questions and eight categories (*domains*) of how tinnitus can be a problem for a person. The eight domains were identified as being the most important areas for evaluating results of treatment for tinnitus. Each domain has its own set of questions within the TFI. The domains are listed below.

1. Emotional reactions
2. Intrusiveness
3. Sleep disturbance
4. Trouble relaxing
5. Hearing difficulties
6. Interference with concentration
7. Reduced sense of control
8. Reduced quality of life

It is my recommendation to use the TFI for assessing outcomes of treatment with TRT. I am, of course, biased because I was one of the investigators who developed the TFI.[17] Regardless of my personal bias, development of the TFI was a rigorous effort, and the questionnaire has attained worldwide recognition (it's been translated into over 20 languages). All that being said, some kind of tinnitus questionnaire should be used to assess the overall effectiveness of treatment. At least a dozen questionnaires have been validated for assessing the impact of tinnitus on a person's life. A few have also been validated for responsiveness.

CHAPTER 3

Patient Categories and Examples of Patients in Each Category

The TRT evaluation provides the essential information to place patients into one of five treatment categories: 0, 1, 2, 3, or 4. Determining the category for an individual patient requires answering four questions: (1) How much does tinnitus impact the person's life? (2) How does the person *perceive the significance* of any hearing loss? (3) Does the person have decreased sound tolerance, and if so, how much of a problem is it? (4) Is there prolonged worsening of the person's condition (tinnitus and/or hyperacusis) following exposure to moderate levels of sound?[19]

Below I will describe each of the five patient categories, along with an example of a patient assigned to each category. The examples are limited to describing how these patients were evaluated, the results of their evaluation, and how they were categorized. The case examples align with Jastreboff's description of TRT.[4,5]

Category 0

Category 0 patients are only minimally bothered by their tinnitus, or they have had their tinnitus for a short period of time.[5,19] They receive an abbreviated version of the TRT counseling, which focuses on learning to think differently about (*reclassify*) tinnitus as a benign or meaningless stimulus, along with advice to enrich their sound environment to optimize habituation to the tinnitus. Ear-level sound generators are not normally recommended. If these patients have hearing difficulties, they should use hearing aids.

> Category 0 patients are only minimally bothered by their tinnitus, or they have had their tinnitus for a short period of time.

Samantha

Samantha is a 36-year-old single mother of two young children. She recently lost her job and has been unable to find new employment. Her situation has left her increasingly depressed, and she often has difficulty even getting out of bed in the morning. One morning, while lying in bed, she noticed a "high-pitched squeal" in her ears. She at first thought it was temporary, especially because she didn't hear it during the day. The sound persisted morning after morning, and she became increasingly concerned about it.

Samantha did not have health insurance, so she went to a warehouse store where hearing aids were sold, hoping someone might know what to do about the sound in her ears. She spoke with a hearing aid dispenser who knew about TRT and referred her to a local audiologist who was trained in TRT. She visited the audiologist, who conducted an interview with her and also tested her hearing.

Following the evaluation, the audiologist told Samantha that she was a TRT category 0 patient. That meant she had essentially normal hearing along with the tinnitus, which was not severe. Although her tinnitus was cause for some concern, she was mostly curious as to what it was and why it was persisting.

Category 1

Category 1 includes patients who have a significant problem with tinnitus.[5] They do not have hyperacusis (a loudness tolerance problem), nor do they report any significant hearing difficulties. They receive the full TRT counseling and are advised to wear ear-level sound generators adjusted to emit constant sound close to but below the mixing point. The sound should be neither annoying nor distracting.

> Category 1 includes patients who have a significant problem with tinnitus.

Rodrigue

Rodrigue is a 57-year-old warehouse worker who unloads trucks and drives a forklift most of the day. He enjoys his work because of its fast pace and was recently promoted to supervisor. His work environment is fairly noisy, mostly due to the forklift. He did not have any difficulties hearing but noticed that his ears were occasionally making a "chirping" sound.

One evening, Rodrigue attended a professional basketball game. People were yelling and screaming, and those close to him seemed to be "screaming right into his ears." When he was at home later that night, his ears made a pronounced sound that he described as "hissing." As a result, he had trouble sleeping that night. The sound persisted, and Rodrigue could not get adequate sleep over the next few weeks. He felt drained, and his fatigue began to negatively affect his job performance.

He made an appointment with an otolaryngologist, who completed a physical examination. The otolaryngologist said "nothing could be done" medically about his tinnitus but that an audiologist in the same office provided tinnitus services. Rodrigue met with the audiologist, who conducted a full TRT evaluation.

The evaluation included completing the TRT Initial Interview, some tinnitus questionnaires, and a comprehensive hearing evaluation. The audiologist sat down with Rodrigue after the evaluation and explained that, based on the results, Rodrigue would be considered a category 1 patient.

Category 2

Category 2 patients are the same as category 1 except they also have significant hearing difficulties. In addition to the full TRT counseling, they wear hearing aids that have a built-in sound generator (known as *combination instruments*). Counseling is modified somewhat to focus on the hearing problems.

> Category 2 patients are the same as category 1 except they also have significant hearing difficulties.

Shelley

Shelley worked as a financial adviser. She had her own office and was well established in her community. As she neared retirement age, she noticed she was having more and more trouble understanding her clients. In addition, she was experiencing a "whining" sound in her ears that seemed to be getting louder. Her hearing and tinnitus problems reached a point where she felt compelled to retire earlier than she had planned.

Following retirement, the tinnitus problem continued to get worse. She made an appointment with an otolaryngologist, who conducted numerous tests. Shelley even had an MRI (magnetic resonance imaging) procedure to see if anything might show up on a brain scan. All of the tests, including the MRI, came back negative, and the otolaryngologist said nothing more could be done. It was suggested that she meet with an audiologist, who could at least help her with her hearing problem.

Shelley was less concerned about her hearing problem because she was no longer meeting with clients. She was, however, experiencing severe reactions to her tinnitus. She thought it "couldn't hurt" to meet with an audiologist to discuss her issues. The audiologist answered many questions about her tinnitus but was unable to provide anything further. The audiologist knew of a physician in another city who offered remote (virtual) counseling. The physician was contacted and agreed to work with Shelley.

The physician asked for additional testing to be done by the audiologist. The audiologist did the additional testing, and the physician took over after that. Shelley and the physician had a Zoom meeting where they spoke face-to-face on their respective computers. The physician asked all the questions on the TRT Initial Interview. Based on the information from the audiologist and the Initial Interview, the physician determined that Shelley was a category 2 patient. That meant that Shelley had significant hearing difficulties and a severe case of bothersome tinnitus that required intervention. She would receive the full TRT counseling and wear hearing aids that have a built-in sound generator.

Category 3

Category 3 patients have hyperacusis (decreased loudness tolerance) as their primary complaint, with or without significant tinnitus.[5] Prior to any intervention for tinnitus, the hyperacusis is treated, which involves a modified version of the TRT counseling along with wearing ear-level sound generators. If the patient also has hearing difficulties, then hearing aids with a built-in sound generator (combination instruments) are used. The TRT protocol for evaluating and treating category 3 patients is described in appendix D.

> Category 3 patients have hyperacusis (decreased loudness tolerance) as their primary complaint, with or without significant tinnitus.

Baz

Baz is a 38-year-old delivery driver. He has been delivering packages for one company for the past nine years. He usually drives with his door open (while seat-belted, of course) so that he can quickly jump in and out of his delivery van. He has therefore been exposed to traffic noise for all these years.

About a year ago the traffic noise became annoying to Baz. He started wearing foam earplugs to block the sound while he was driving. He also realized he had tinnitus, which was most noticeable when he wore the earplugs. He eventually was wearing earplugs all day at work, and he even started wearing them whenever he was outdoors or driving his personal car.

One day, while delivering a package to an audiology office, Baz spoke with the audiologist about his ear problems. The audiologist happened to be trained in TRT and offered to do an evaluation. They scheduled an appointment.

Baz had a complete evaluation by the audiologist. His hearing was not a problem, so he did not need hearing aids. His tinnitus was mildly bothersome and only required some minimal counseling. He was diagnosed as having a severe case of hyperacusis, which was the reason he was so dependent on wearing earplugs. The audiologist explained that traffic noise is so loud as to potentially be damaging to the ears. This was very likely the reason Baz had both tinnitus and hyperacusis. The hyperacusis diagnosis meant that he was a TRT category 3 patient.

Category 4

Category 4 patients have prolonged worsening (exacerbation) of their tinnitus and/or their hyperacusis—the exacerbation is caused by exposure to certain sounds. By definition, the worsening lasts until at least the next morning. If hyperacusis is the main problem, then the hyperacusis treatment is used as for category 3 patients. Otherwise, treatment focuses on tinnitus as for category 1 patients. Category 4 patients may be the most difficult to treat successfully.[20,21] An explanation of how category 4 patients are evaluated and treated with TRT is provided in appendix E.

> Category 4 patients have prolonged worsening (exacerbation) of their tinnitus and/or their hyperacusis—the exacerbation is caused by exposure to certain sounds.

Marcus

Marcus was in the military for 20 years and then worked as an accountant for another 20 years until he retired. In the military, he served on carrier ships and was often on the flight deck. He was trained to protect his ears while on the flight deck because of the extremely high noise made by jet engines. In spite of his use of earplugs and earmuffs, he experienced hearing loss, which was very noticeable during his years as an accountant.

Marcus also experienced tinnitus, which he described as his "birdies." As long as he was working, he was able to ignore the tinnitus most of the time. When he retired, however, he had a lot of idle time, and he paid more and more attention to his tinnitus. At some point, he became so obsessed with his tinnitus that he went to a psychiatrist at his local medical center that served military Veterans. The psychiatrist did not know much about tinnitus, and she prescribed medication to help him relax.

Marcus had previously received ongoing services from audiologists at the medical center. They provided him with hearing aids. He knew that one of the audiologists specialized in tinnitus management. He met with this audiologist and learned about TRT. She had received full TRT training some years previously from Drs. Pawel and Margaret Jastreboff and had since provided TRT to over a hundred Veterans who had severe tinnitus.

During the appointment, the audiologist focused on understanding Marcus's tinnitus problem. She already had a record of his hearing loss and his experience wearing hearing aids. All she really needed to do was to ask the questions from the TRT Initial Interview, which she did. She learned how Marcus was severely affected by his tinnitus. She also discovered that he had a particular type of tinnitus that would place him in TRT category 4.

Category 4 means that certain sounds (not just loud sounds) cause tinnitus to become noticeably more intense. If Marcus sat next to someone in a restaurant, and that person spoke into his ear, his tinnitus seemed to flare up. Further, the tinnitus stayed louder until at least the following day. These symptoms describe TRT category 4, which is reserved for patients whose tinnitus becomes more intense when exposed to certain sounds, like Marcus reported, and stays louder for at least another day. Category 4 patients are fairly uncommon, and they are thought to pose the greatest challenges for tinnitus management relative to the other treatment categories.[20,21]

CHAPTER 4

Walking You Through the Tinnitus and Hearing Survey

Although this book is focused on TRT, my research over the years has led me to modify the TRT protocol somewhat to provide what I believe is the best tinnitus care. In this chapter I will note where I am inserting modifications that are not "officially" part of TRT as described by the primary founder of TRT, Dr. Pawel Jastreboff.[4,5] The remaining chapters are mostly consistent with the protocol espoused by Jastreboff and Hazell (2004).[4]

The remainder of this book involves role modeling of me, your TRT clinician, speaking directly to you, a patient seeking help for bothersome tinnitus. In this chapter you will complete the *Tinnitus and Hearing Survey*. In chapter 5, I will explain each question on the TRT Initial Interview—why each question is important, the results of our fictional evaluation, and how different results might indicate differences in how someone would be categorized for treatment purposes. At that point we will have all the information we need to know how to go about treatment. Chapter 6 covers how sound therapy is used specifically with TRT. Chapter 7 is a counseling session to describe background information that is helpful for understanding the TRT neurophysiological model. Chapter 8 continues the counseling to explain the neurophysiological model, which is the foundation of TRT.

Ready? Here we go.

Welcome to Your First TRT Visit

Welcome! And thank you for coming into my clinic today. I understand you have tinnitus and that it is greatly bothering you. I specialize in Tinnitus Retraining Therapy (TRT), which was introduced by Dr. Pawel Jastreboff around 1990 and is used around the world. Before we start your assessment, let's talk about what we're trying to accomplish.

Primary Tinnitus

Some people confuse their tinnitus with different types of ear and head noises. You have described your tinnitus as being *constant* and that you can hear it in almost any situation. You also said you have had tinnitus for more than six months, which means your tinnitus is *persistent*.[14] I'm glad that you met with an otolaryngologist who ruled out any medical conditions that might be causing your tinnitus. It is therefore clear that you have *primary* tinnitus, which may be thought of as "hyperactivity of the brain's auditory nervous system."[3]

Tinnitus and Hearing Difficulties

You mentioned that you have trouble hearing, and you are concerned that your tinnitus is causing your hearing problems. We will first start with that concern. People who have tinnitus usually have some degree of hearing loss, and many also have decreased sound tolerance—usually hyperacusis, which is defined as reduced tolerance to the loudness of sound.[22] It is therefore essential for this evaluation to include an assessment of how well you hear, how you are affected by your tinnitus, and whether you have decreased sound tolerance.

> People who have tinnitus usually have some degree of hearing loss...

The Tinnitus and Hearing Survey

[Note that the Tinnitus and Hearing Survey is not part of TRT as described by Dr. Jastreboff.[5] It is added here because it addresses the need to ensure that tinnitus is not being blamed for any hearing problems. It also serves to screen for a sound tolerance problem. It takes only a couple of minutes to complete and provides valuable information.]

We will start by having you complete the Tinnitus and Hearing Survey (Fig. 4-1).[23] The survey has three sections: Tinnitus, Hearing, and Sound Tolerance. Each section contains statements that refer to problems you might be experiencing with these auditory conditions. Read each statement and indicate whether it is "not a problem" or if it is a "small," "moderate," "big," or "very big" problem. This should only take you about two minutes to complete.

Tinnitus and Hearing Survey

	No, **not** a problem	Yes, a **small** problem	Yes, a **moderate** problem	Yes, a **big** problem	Yes, a **very big** problem	
A Tinnitus						
Over the last week, tinnitus kept me from sleeping.	0	1	2	3	4	
Over the last week, tinnitus kept me from concentrating on reading.	0	1	2	3	4	
Over the last week, tinnitus kept me from relaxing.	0	1	2	3	4	**Grand Total**
Over the last week, I couldn' t get my mind off of my tinnitus.	0	1	2	3	4	
	___	___	___	___	___	[ ]
			Total of each column			
B. Hearing						
Over the last week, I couldn't understand what others were saying in noisy or crowded places.	0	1	2	3	4	
Over the last week, I couldn't understand what people were saying on TV or in movies.	0	1	2	3	4	
Over the last week, I couldn't understand people with soft voices.	0	1	2	3	4	**Grand Total**
Over the last week, I couldn't understand what was being said in group conversations.	0	1	2	3	4	
	___	___	___	___	___	[ ]
			Total of each column			
C. Sound Tolerance						
Over the last week, sounds were too loud or uncomfortable for me when they seemed normal to others around me.*	0	1	2	3	4	

If you responded l, 2, 3, or 4 to the statement above:

Please list two examples of sounds that are too loud or uncomfortable for you, but seem normal to others: _____

*If sounds are too loud for you while wearing hearing aids, please tell your audiologist. _____

For office use only (II): ☐ M ☐ H ☐ NS ☐ P ☐ N

Full size survey can be downloaded at: **https://earsgonewrong.org/resources-tinnitus-hearing-survey/** Or use your phone on the QR code —>

> **4-1. The Tinnitus and Hearing Survey.** The Tinnitus and Hearing Survey is used to determine how much of a problem a person has with tinnitus and with hearing loss.[23] The survey is designed so that any problems with tinnitus are not confused with hearing problems. Likewise, any problems with hearing are not conflated with tinnitus. Section C screens for a problem tolerating sound, which often occurs along with tinnitus.

Thank you for completing the Tinnitus and Hearing Survey. I need to tell you why I had you complete this little form. I already mentioned that people who have tinnitus usually also have some degree of hearing loss. Tinnitus is obvious—you can hear it. With hearing loss, only its effects are noticed—generally, difficulty hearing in some situations.

> Tinnitus is obvious—you can hear it. With hearing loss, only its effects are noticed...

Does Tinnitus Make It Difficult to Hear?

For someone with both tinnitus and hearing difficulties, it would be natural to blame the tinnitus for the hearing problems.[24] In such cases, a hearing evaluation will usually reveal some amount of hearing loss. More specifically, the hearing evaluation reveals a *loss of hearing sensitivity*. With hearing loss, sound has to be louder before it can be heard compared to the average young person with "normal" hearing sensitivity. The hearing difficulties are due to the hearing loss—not the tinnitus.

Hearing Loss Explained

We can hear a range of frequencies (or *pitches*)—think of the keys on a piano keyboard, with low pitches toward the left side gradually progressing to high pitches toward the right. Human speech consists of low-frequency vowel sounds ("a, e, i, o, u, and sometimes y") and high-frequency consonant sounds, such as "th," "sh," "f," and "s." Vowels are louder (high-energy) sounds, and consonants are softer (low-energy) sounds. It is critical to hear the low-energy consonants in order to understand speech clearly.

Hearing loss usually starts in the high-frequency range—where the consonants are. When there is background noise, such as in a restaurant, the soft consonant sounds are naturally covered up (*masked*) by the noise. The vowels are heard, but the consonants are missing. That's why it's difficult to hear speech when there is background noise.

Imagine trying to distinguish between "cat" and "cap" if you can't hear "t" or "p." Or how about hearing "thread" and thinking the word is "bread"? Other examples: "nice" and "mice," "first" and "thirst," "sheep" and "sleep." The list is endless. The jokes are endless too, but they make the point: "What kind is it?" "Twelve thirty." Or the cartoon with three elderly gentlemen: Person 1: "It's windy today." Person 2: "No, it's Thursday." Person 3: "So am I! Let's have a beer!"

> The point is that hearing difficulties are caused by hearing loss and not by tinnitus.

Hearing loss is complex, and this explanation addresses what is typically experienced by a person who has hearing loss. The point is that hearing difficulties are caused by hearing loss and not by tinnitus. Let's review your responses on the Tinnitus and Hearing Survey.

Your Responses on the Tinnitus and Hearing Survey

(Please refer to Fig. 4-1.) For Section A (the Tinnitus section), you said that, because of your tinnitus, sleep is a "very big" problem, and that concentrating, relaxing, and keeping your mind off your tinnitus are all "big" problems. When we score these responses on a scale from 0 to 4, sleep is 4, and your other three "big" problems are each 3. Your total score for the Tinnitus section is 13 (out of a possible maximum 16 points).

Let's do the same thing with Section B (Hearing). You said understanding speech in noisy situations is a "big" problem (score = 3). Understanding speech on TV and in movies is a "small" problem (score = 1). Understanding people with soft voices is a "moderate" problem (score = 2), and understanding people in group conversations is a "big" problem (score = 3). Therefore, your total score for the Hearing section is 9 (out of a possible maximum 16 points).

For Section C (Sound Tolerance), you indicated sounds being too loud or uncomfortable for you are a "small" problem. Because of this response, you were then asked to complete the next item that says to list examples of the kinds of sounds that bother you. The examples you listed were "dishes" and "children's voices."

So how do we interpret your responses on the Tinnitus and Hearing Survey? Your score on the Tinnitus section indicates that your tinnitus is significantly impacting your life. Your score on the Hearing section indicates that hearing is also a significant problem, but maybe not to the same degree as your tinnitus problem. You reported a "small" sound tolerance problem along with some examples, so that's something we will need to explore further.

How Might Others Respond on the Tinnitus and Hearing Survey?

People who blame their tinnitus for their hearing difficulties will typically have a low score on the Tinnitus section and a high score on the Hearing section. They thought they had a tinnitus problem, but they really had a hearing problem. In such a case there may be no need for further tinnitus services, but the hearing problem may need to be addressed with hearing aids.

There are no cutoff scores on the Tinnitus and Hearing Survey, meaning there are no division points between a mild, moderate, or severe problem. The survey is a tool to assist in separating hearing problems from tinnitus problems and to screen for a sound tolerance problem. It generally does a good job with each, but it should be used along with a medical history and hearing evaluation. The information obtained from the survey, medical history, and hearing evaluation is usually sufficient to determine whether special services are needed for the tinnitus, if hearing loss is a concern warranting the use of hearing aids, and if there is a problem tolerating sound.

CHAPTER 5

Walking You Through the TRT Initial Interview

Because your tinnitus clearly is a problem for you (and not being blamed for your hearing difficulties), the next thing we will do is complete the TRT Initial Interview.[11,25] This interview was designed to describe problems with tinnitus, hearing loss, and sound intolerance. Since you do not have a problem with sound intolerance, we will just focus on the sections of the TRT Initial Interview that address tinnitus and hearing. Some of the questions are similar to those that would be asked as part of your medical history (described in appendix B).

As an aside, it should be mentioned that different clinicians will interview patients in different ways, while covering the same areas that are essential in TRT. What's important is that the form we're using addresses all of the topics that are critical to determining how tinnitus affects *you* and how treatment might be modified to address your individual concerns. Reading each question word for word ensures that the questions are asked in a standardized manner. That is what we're now going to do.

TRT Initial Interview

The first series includes 18 questions that are specific to your tinnitus.[11] Answer these questions thinking about your tinnitus *over the last month*. The first four questions ask you to describe characteristics of the *sound* of your tinnitus (not any reactions to, or effects of, tinnitus).

Questions 1 and 2. Where is the location of your tinnitus (head, right ear, left ear, both ears)? Is your tinnitus louder on one side of your head than the other?

These first two questions address the concern that your tinnitus might be perceived in only one ear or one side of the head (*unilateral* tinnitus) or that it might be more prominent in one ear than the other or in one side of the head than the other (*asymmetric* tinnitus). As explained in appendix B, unilateral or asymmetric tinnitus might indicate the need for a physical examination and an assessment by an audiologist to rule out a tumor or other abnormality.[14,26,27]

You responded that your tinnitus sounds about the same in both ears. You have also been examined by an otolaryngologist, so we are reasonably certain that there are no underlying medical concerns.

Question 3. Is your tinnitus a constant sound or an intermittent sound?

You have described your tinnitus as constant, meaning you can always or usually hear it in any quiet environment.[28,29] Intermittent tinnitus, however, is not so straightforward. People can have sounds in their ears or head that come and go.

My definition for tinnitus is "sound in the ears or head that lasts at least five minutes and occurs at least every week."[3] If the sound lasts less than five minutes, or not as often as every week, then it is a different form of ear noise.[28,29] For example, *transient ear noise* (fleeting tinnitus) is a sudden tonal sound in one ear that may be experienced along with a sense of ear fullness and hearing loss. All of these symptoms resolve within a few minutes. This is normal and experienced by almost everyone.

There is also *temporary ear noise* that can follow exposure to loud sound (such as a rock concert or construction noise). Temporary ear noise (or *temporary tinnitus*) should be noticed as a red flag to protect the ears from loud sound.

> Temporary ear noise (or *temporary tinnitus*) should be noticed as a red flag to protect the ears from loud sound.

Question 4. Does your tinnitus fluctuate in volume (that is, does the volume change *on its own*)?

You responded that the volume of your tinnitus seems to fluctuate by being louder on some days and softer on others.

That kind of fluctuation would be expected for just about anyone with tinnitus. The main concern here is that the tinnitus fluctuations occur randomly and spontaneously and are not the result of exposure to certain kinds of sounds, which is a special concern that is addressed in question 8.

Question 5. Please describe the onset of your tinnitus (gradual or sudden). When did it start?

There is a lot to unpack in this question. It is intended to determine two things: First, what event or events might be responsible for triggering your tinnitus in the first place? Second, how long have you had tinnitus (its duration)?

Why is it important to know what might be responsible for triggering your tinnitus? In general, the circumstances surrounding the onset of your tinnitus can make a difference in how you react to it. Those circumstances can include being exposed to loud sound caused by some activity that you enjoy (such as listening to loud music, hunting with a rifle, or racing motorcycles) or that you *don't* enjoy (such as daily factory noise, a firecracker going off close to one ear, or being blasted with an air horn at close range). Your tinnitus might have started in the hospital when you were fighting a serious illness. It might have started following a car accident or when you were exposed to an explosion. It might

> ...the circumstances surrounding the onset of your tinnitus can make a difference in how you react to it.

have started during a particularly stressful situation. And it might have started out of the blue for no known reason. These varied circumstances would cause different degrees of trauma, anywhere from "no trauma" to "extreme trauma." The more traumatic the event, the more likely the tinnitus will trigger memories of it. This can result in a vicious circle of thinking about the tinnitus, remembering the traumatic event, reacting emotionally to the memory, and thinking about the tinnitus. This repeat cycle of awareness → memories → anxiety → awareness describes why many people stay stuck being distressed by their tinnitus.

Why is it important to know *how long* you've had tinnitus? It's a fairly arbitrary distinction, but according to the AAO-HNSF, tinnitus that has been experienced for less than six months is considered *recent-onset,* while tinnitus that has been experienced for at least six months is considered *persistent.*[14] Their rationale for making this distinction is that most research studies evaluating treatments for tinnitus require that participants have experienced tinnitus for at least six months to be reasonably sure that the tinnitus is stable. Supporting their rationale is a study that showed that recent-onset

> ...tinnitus that has been experienced for less than six months is considered recent-onset, while tinnitus that has been experienced for at least six months is considered persistent.

tinnitus is more likely than persistent tinnitus to reduce in intensity or even disappear altogether.[30] The AAO-HNSF further noted that people whose tinnitus was still bothersome after six months were more likely to require treatment than those whose tinnitus had been bothersome for less than six months.[14]

You responded that your tinnitus started gradually with your long-term noise exposure at work. The work noise was annoying to you, and thinking about your tinnitus reminds you of the unpleasant noise, along with what you felt was a hostile work environment. You became increasingly aware of your tinnitus, and it also seemed that the tinnitus became louder and more continuous. Your circumstances appear to be a textbook case for why your tinnitus is so bothersome to you.

Question 6. What does your *most bothersome* tinnitus sound like?

At a major tinnitus clinic with records from thousands of patients, about half of the patients described their tinnitus as consisting of a single sound while the other half described it as consisting of multiple sounds.[31] It is important to identify the tinnitus sound that is the most bothersome. If there is only one sound, then that sound is described to answer this question. If it is more than one sound, then we need to identify which of the different sounds is the most bothersome, for a number of reasons.

First, we need to know which tinnitus sound is the most bothersome to focus

...we need to know which tinnitus sound is the most bothersome to focus treatment on habituating (stop reacting) to that particular sound.

WALKING YOU THROUGH THE TRT INITIAL INTERVIEW

treatment on habituating (stop reacting) to that particular sound. Second, if you will be using wearable ear-level sound generators, the sound of those generators will be adjusted relative to your most bothersome tinnitus. Third, we will evaluate your tinnitus using procedures to match your tinnitus to sounds that you will hear through earphones. The matching needs to be done to your most bothersome tinnitus.

You have described your tinnitus as consisting of two sounds—one is dominant and the other is barely noticeable. Your dominant tinnitus sounds like a "high-pitched squealing sound." Your second sound is a soft, low-pitched "hum." We will be focusing on the dominant sound for the remainder of this evaluation and for treatment.

It should be noted that, as a natural consequence of habituating to your most bothersome tinnitus, you typically habituate to *all* of your tinnitus. You can think of this phenomenon as habituating to tinnitus *as a concept* rather than to just one sound.

> ...as a natural consequence of habituating to your most bothersome tinnitus, you typically habituate to *all* of your tinnitus.

Question 7. Do you have "bad days" when your tinnitus is more bothersome than usual, or does it seem equally bothersome from day to day? *If yes*, how often do you have these bad days?

Some people will respond that every day is a bad day because of their tinnitus. That's generally true for anyone who has bothersome tinnitus. The point of this question, however, is to determine whether some days are *particularly difficult* because of the tinnitus, and if so, what might be responsible for those bad days.

Most likely, a person's bad day is due to an unusually high level of psychological or emotional stress. Stress in general is a contributor to tinnitus distress, although it is also true that tinnitus causes stress.[32] This chicken-or-the-egg relationship between tinnitus and stress can only be evaluated on an individual basis to determine the degree to which stressful events contribute to tinnitus being bothersome versus how much tinnitus contributes to feeling stressed.[33] Regardless, it is important to identify events that are stress-inducing. Treatment should address these stressful events by attempting to reduce or eliminate their impact. Evaluation and treatment by a behavioral health provider might be helpful. (Note that some audiologists fit the ear-level devices and then send their patients to psychologists—calling the whole process TRT.)

> Stress in general is a contributor to tinnitus distress, although it is also true that tinnitus causes stress.

The same chicken-or-the-egg question pertains to stress and the *perceived loudness* of tinnitus. Some people report that their tinnitus "spikes" on certain days, meaning the tinnitus becomes louder and consequently more bothersome. The spiking is often associated with stressful events. Many studies have shown that the perceived loudness of a person's tinnitus often corresponds with how bothersome it is.[34-36]

> ...the perceived loudness of a person's tinnitus often corresponds with how bothersome it is.

You reported that you have bad days when your tinnitus seems especially loud and bothersome. These bad days are often related to your interpersonal relationships when you are dealing with conflict. You normally avoid conflict because you know it makes you feel stressed. It is occasionally unavoidable, and when it happens you become more aware of, and more annoyed by, your tinnitus. Dealing with difficult interpersonal relationships may require special assistance from a psychologist or other behavioral health provider.

Question 8. Do sounds ever cause a change in the loudness of your tinnitus? *If louder,* **what kinds of sounds cause this change? When any of these sounds cause your tinnitus to change, how long does the change last? When you hear a sound that causes your tinnitus to change, does the effect sometimes last until the next morning after you've slept?** *If yes,* **what kinds of sounds cause this to happen?**

This is a critical series of questions to help determine whether you would be placed in a special TRT category (chapter 3). The concern is whether exposure to certain low-level sounds causes a prolonged worsening (exacerbation) of your tinnitus. If the worsening lasts at least until the next day, then you would most likely be a TRT category 4 patient. Patients in this category are relatively uncommon and are also the most difficult to treat successfully.[4,20,21]

You noted that sometimes your tinnitus does become louder as a result of exposure to certain sounds. After further questioning we determined that the sounds you are referring to are loud enough to cause damage to your ears. That would be a concern for anyone, and I strongly recommend protecting your ears with earplugs or earmuffs whenever you are around such sounds. It appears, however, that low-level sounds do not cause prolonged worsening of your tinnitus, and so you would not be considered a TRT category 4 patient.

WALKING YOU THROUGH THE TRT INITIAL INTERVIEW

Question 9. Do you use ear protection (earplugs or earmuffs)? *If yes*, **why do you use ear protection? (☐To keep tinnitus from getting louder; ☐Trouble tolerating everyday sounds that seem normal to others; ☐Other reason_____) Do you use it specifically because of the tinnitus?** *If so*, **what percent of the time do you use earplugs or earmuffs** *for your tinnitus*? **Do you use earplugs or earmuffs** *for your tinnitus* **when it's fairly quiet?**

When I attended my first TRT training seminar back in 1997, I learned something that was a real eye-opener to me. Before the seminar I had had tinnitus for about 20 years, and I also was dealing with hyperacusis (intolerance to the loudness of sounds that most people can tolerate comfortably). My solution was to wear earplugs, which reduced the loudness of sound to a comfortable level. I found that the more I wore earplugs, the more I *needed* to wear earplugs. Little did I know that what I was doing was making my hyperacusis worse. During the seminar I learned that I was *overprotecting* my ears, which was making me more sensitive, and less tolerant, to the loudness of everyday sounds.

> ...the more I wore earplugs, the more I needed to wear earplugs.

In your case, you have not been using ear protection at all, much less in the manner that I was using it. I already advised you to use earplugs or earmuffs whenever you are around sound that seems loud enough to damage your ears. This should be the only time you use hearing protection. Any other use of hearing protection, such as what I was doing, would mean you are overprotecting your ears.

If you're interested in knowing more about why over-protecting your ears can be a problem, I'll briefly describe a relevant study. This study compared what happened to people when sound was added (wearing ear-level sound generators) for two weeks compared to reducing sound (wearing earplugs) for two weeks.[37] Wearing the sound generators resulted in a *greater* ability to tolerate the loudness of sounds. Wearing earplugs resulted in a *reduced* ability to tolerate the loudness of sounds. This same outcome has been observed in other studies.[38-40] The effect has implications for both hyperacusis and tinnitus. I have written about it, if you want to learn more.[3,41]

Question 10. Are you currently receiving any other treatment specifically for your tinnitus? If yes, what?

There are all kinds of different treatments for tinnitus. I have written about various methods, and I noted four that are well established and based on clinical and research evidence.[3,42] One of those four methods is TRT. The others are cognitive behavioral therapy (CBT), Tinnitus Activities Treatment, and Progressive Tinnitus Management. Although unlikely, it's possible you are receiving CBT from a psychologist while you are receiving TRT. That would be acceptable as long as your care is coordinated between providers.

There are countless pills (nutritional supplements) and sound therapy programs promoted on the internet for treating tinnitus. None of the pills have been shown to be beneficial for tinnitus so they are basically a waste of money. Sound therapy refers to any use of sound to reduce effects of tinnitus. With TRT you will be counseled to "enrich your sound environment 24/7," so if you are using sound therapy, that would be acceptable along with TRT. I would suggest you use sounds that are

> Sound therapy refers to any use of sound to reduce effects of tinnitus.

either free or very low cost. We also don't want anything you're using for sound therapy to conflict with what is recommended for TRT. We'll have a lot more to say about sound therapy later.

There are also prescription medications that are used to treat anxiety, depression, and insomnia. These conditions may or may not be caused by the tinnitus. Use of these medications is under the supervision of a physician, and any changes should first be authorized by your physician.

Question 11. What is the *biggest reason* your tinnitus is a problem (not including trouble hearing or trouble understanding speech)?

This question can be rephrased, "What part of your life is most affected by your tinnitus?" Effects of tinnitus on a person's life (*functional* effects) are most typically sleep problems, concentration difficulties, and emotional reactions.[1,43] Reducing or eliminating these effects is the objective of treatment. A reduction in tinnitus awareness is a most welcome consequence of reducing these functional effects.

The question specifically excludes trouble hearing or trouble understanding speech. When you completed the

> Effects of tinnitus on a person's life (functional effects) are most typically sleep problems, concentration difficulties, and emotional reactions.

Tinnitus and Hearing Survey (chapter 4), it addressed the concern that some people feel that their tinnitus causes hearing difficulties. We made sure you understood that hearing difficulties are due to hearing loss and not to tinnitus.

You responded that the main reason tinnitus is a problem for you is because it keeps you awake at night. Your sleep deprivation has gone on for weeks, and you feel tired and irritable all the time. It has affected every aspect of your life. We will make improving your sleep the number one priority of treatment.

> **Question 12. I'm going to read through a list of activities, and I want you to tell me how often your tinnitus keeps you from doing these activities, or how often it negatively affects these activities in any way. Please don't include trouble hearing or trouble understanding speech when you answer these questions.**

We just asked in question 11, what is the *biggest reason* your tinnitus is a problem? We're now expanding on that open-ended question to ask about life activities that are commonly reported to be affected by tinnitus. We want to know how much any of these activities have been affected by your tinnitus or if an activity is irrelevant (not applicable—N/A).

	Never	Rarely	Some-times	Often	Always	N/A
Concentration?	☐	☐	☐	☐	☐	☐
Sleep?	☐	☐	☐	☐	☐	☐
Quiet resting activities (reading, relaxing, etc.)?	☐	☐	☐	☐	☐	☐
Work? (select N/A if retired)	☐	☐	☐	☐	☐	☐
Day-to-day responsibilities outside of work?	☐	☐	☐	☐	☐	☐
Going to restaurants?	☐	☐	☐	☐	☐	☐
Participating in or observing sports events?	☐	☐	☐	☐	☐	☐
Social activities?	☐	☐	☐	☐	☐	☐
Anything else?	☐	☐	☐	☐	☐	☐

Consistent with your previous answer (question 11), your sleep has "often" been affected. You also reported that concentration, work, and social activities are "sometimes" affected by your tinnitus. Getting better sleep every night should help with these other effects of your tinnitus.

In addition to knowing how tinnitus affects you so that we can focus the treatment accordingly, your responses to these questions serve as *baseline* (before-treatment) measures to compare to during

...your responses to these questions serve as baseline (before-treatment) measures to compare to during and following treatment.

and following treatment. This will help us to know if the treatment is effective in reducing the functional effects of tinnitus on your life.

Question 13. What percent of your *total awake time*, over the last month, were you *noticing or thinking about* your tinnitus? Please give an average percentage over the last month.

Question 14. What percent of your *total awake time*, over the last month, were you *annoyed, distressed, or irritated* by your tinnitus? Please give an average percentage over the last month.

Questions 13 and 14 are similar and may be the most important questions with respect to the overall intent of TRT, which is habituation—a form of subconscious learning to stop being aware of, and stop reacting to, tinnitus.

Question 13 asks how much time you spend *thinking about* (or being aware of) your tinnitus. The question is therefore specific to *habituation of tinnitus perception*.

Question 14 asks how much of your time you are *annoyed, distressed, or irritated* by your tinnitus, which addresses *habituation of tinnitus reactions* (*reactions* refers to these negative emotions).

> Habituation of both the perception of and reactions to tinnitus would tell us TRT has been successful.

Habituation of both the perception of and reactions to tinnitus would tell us TRT has been successful.[44-46] This would be seen by the percentages of your time *aware of* and *reacting to* tinnitus dropping substantially from your pre-treatment numbers.

You responded that during your total awake time, you have been aware of your tinnitus about 70% of the time and have also been annoyed, distressed, or irritated by your tinnitus about 70% of the time. What that means is, anytime you think about your tinnitus it causes emotional reactions. We are going to do everything we can to get those percentages down as much as possible.

The next three questions (15, 16, and 17) all ask you to choose a number on a scale of zero to ten to indicate how much your tinnitus affects you. These questions are also important to determine how well TRT works for you. The numbers you provide now will be your baseline numbers that reflect how much of a problem your tinnitus is before receiving treatment. Following treatment, we should see those numbers go down—the closer to zero the better. Let's first discuss the intent of each question, and then you can choose the number for each question that you feel is the most accurate in describing your tinnitus.

> **Question 15. How *strong*, or *loud*, was your tinnitus, on average, over the last month? "0" would be "no tinnitus"; "10" would be "as loud as you can imagine."**

The loudness of a person's tinnitus cannot be measured objectively. That is, we have no way to accurately quantify how loud a person's tinnitus is on any scale. We can measure the intensity of sounds in the environment using a decibel meter. In fact, using a decibel meter is

> ...we have no way to accurately quantify how loud a person's tinnitus is on any scale.

how we can tell if sound is so loud as to potentially cause damage to the ears.

This question can be difficult to answer because so many people equate the loudness of their tinnitus with how much it bothers them.[36,47] They may think the tinnitus is louder when it is more bothersome and not as loud when it's less bothersome. It's possible that the loudness is actually changing, but that cannot be verified using any type of measuring equipment. A more realistic response would be to not only choose a number from zero to ten but also to mention some sound in the environment that is about the same loudness as the tinnitus.

> **Question 16. How much has tinnitus *annoyed you*, on average, over the last month—not including annoyance from trouble hearing or trouble understanding speech? "0" would be "not annoying at all"; "10" would be "as annoying as you can imagine."**

This question is specific in asking how much your tinnitus has bothered you *emotionally*, which is what *reactions* refers to—annoyance, distress, and irritation. It's another way of asking question 14, "What percent of your *total awake time*, over the last month, were you *annoyed, distressed, or irritated* by your tinnitus?" The main goal of treatment with

> The main goal of treatment with TRT is to facilitate habituation of reactions to tinnitus, which leads automatically to habituation of the perception of tinnitus.

TRT is to facilitate habituation of reactions to tinnitus, which leads automatically to habituation of the perception of tinnitus.[4,5]

> ## Question 17. How much did tinnitus *impact your life*, on average, over the last month—not including impact from trouble hearing or trouble understanding speech? "0" would be "not at all"; "10" would be "as much as you can imagine."

This is really a quality-of-life question and so it could be asked, "How much did tinnitus *reduce your quality of life*, on average, over the last month?" The question is not specific to any particular effects of tinnitus but rather is asking about your life in general and how it is affected (impacted) by your tinnitus.

We've discussed the intent of these last three questions, 15, 16, and 17, and it's time to choose a number on a scale of zero to ten to respond to each one. For question 15, "How *strong*, or *loud*, was your tinnitus . . . ?" you chose "8." You said you were tempted to choose a "10," but you realized that your tinnitus is not "as loud as you can imagine," which would refer to sounds in the environment that you know are louder than your tinnitus.

For question 16, "How much has tinnitus *annoyed* you . . . ?" you chose a "9." That means that tinnitus has severely affected you emotionally. You also chose a "9" for question 17, "How much did tinnitus *impact your life* . . . ?" which is not surprising given your other responses.

Question 18. Do you have any other comments about your tinnitus?

We've covered a lot of territory with the last 17 questions. Question 18 gives you the opportunity to say anything else about your tinnitus that may have been missed or overlooked.

You noted that you have struggled with knowing there is no cure for tinnitus—there are only methods for managing it. You don't feel confident that any form of treatment can help you live a normal life while the tinnitus is still in your head. I completely understand your concern, which is very commonly expressed by people in the same situation. I have, however, seen these people get back on their feet as a result of treatment to the point that tinnitus became a negligible concern in their lives. They learned to habituate to their tinnitus. This may seem overly optimistic, but it's a fact that proper treatment can help the majority of people—to different degrees because everyone has a unique set of circumstances. What matters is meeting with a professional who is trained and experienced in providing tinnitus services and who has your best interests at heart. You also need to do your part to comply with the treatment protocol to the best of your ability.

> ...proper treatment can help the majority of people—to different degrees because everyone has a unique set of circumstances.

We've completed the Tinnitus portion of the TRT Initial Interview. The next series of questions pertains to your ability to tolerate sound. According to the Tinnitus and Hearing Survey, your responses indicated you have a "small" sound tolerance problem. We can explore that further now, starting with question 19.

> ## Question 19. Are sounds bothersome or unpleasant to you when they seem normal to other people around you? *If yes*, what kinds of sounds are bothersome or unpleasant?

It is important that you clearly understand the intent of this question because your response will determine whether or not you are identified as having a problem with sound tolerance. If so, you might be placed in TRT category 3. If not, the remaining questions in this sound tolerance section will be skipped over. The main concern is to determine whether you have trouble tolerating everyday sounds that are tolerated comfortably by the average person.

Your response to this question was "no," so we are done with this section. If you're interested in seeing the sound tolerance questions, the TRT Initial Interview is available online as a free download, and each question is explained, including the questions from the Sound Tolerance section (https://www.rehab.research.va.gov/jour/03/40/2/pdf/Henry.pdf).[11] Also, appendix D in this book describes in detail how a person would be evaluated with the

> The main concern is to determine whether you have trouble tolerating everyday sounds that are tolerated comfortably by the average person.

> The point of these questions about hearing is to determine *how you feel about your hearing*, regardless of the results of your audiogram.

Sound Tolerance section of the Initial Interview and how treatment would be done.

We will now skip ahead to the three questions (31, 32, and 33) about your hearing. Afterward, we will measure your *hearing thresholds* (the softest sounds you can hear) with an audiometer, but the results of that testing (your audiogram) may not agree with your own feelings about how well you hear.[48-50] Some people have substantial hearing loss according to their audiogram but don't feel they have a significant hearing problem. Other people complain about significant hearing difficulties even though their audiogram reveals normal hearing or only a mild hearing loss. The point of these questions about hearing is to determine *how you feel about your hearing,* regardless of the results of your audiogram. Your responses will determine whether you should be placed in category 2, which would suggest that hearing aids would be beneficial as part of your treatment.

Question 31. Do you think you have a hearing problem?

Our ability to hear is most important with respect to understanding what people say (their speech). Hearing speech and understanding speech are two different things. We may hear someone talking but not understand what they're saying. Maybe we understand some words, but we don't understand others.

Difficulty understanding speech is usually first noticed when there is background noise, which was explained when you completed the Tinnitus and Hearing Survey (see the section "Hearing Loss Explained" in chapter

> ...a person's ability to understand speech relies on the entire auditory system— from the cochlea up through the brain.

4). There is much more to the story, however, because understanding speech relies on areas of the brain that process speech signals. This is a complex topic, but the bottom line is, a person's ability to understand speech relies on the entire auditory system—from the cochlea up through the brain. Any of these areas can affect how well you understand speech (as well as other sounds).

One more thing to be aware of: I described the difference between hearing and understanding speech. We also have to be able to *listen* to speech, which requires paying attention to what is being said. A person with tinnitus might have the ability to hear well and understand well yet have difficulty listening because the tinnitus is so distracting.

We know that you have difficulty understanding speech because of your responses on the Tinnitus and Hearing Survey. Because of that difficulty, amplification (hearing aids) would most likely be helpful for you.

Question 32. Have you ever worn hearing aids?

Although you have significant a problem with your hearing, you have never worn hearing aids.

Question 33. Have you ever had hearing aids recommended to you?

You have never had a hearing test, and you have never had hearing aids recommended to you. Because of your hearing problems, we will most likely recommend that you start wearing hearing aids.

Question 34. How much of a problem is *tinnitus* (if you are not including problems from trouble hearing or trouble understanding speech)? "0" would be "no problem at all"; "10" would be "as much as you can imagine."

You rated your tinnitus problem as a "9."

Question 35. How much of a problem is *trouble tolerating sound*? "0" would be "no problem at all"; "10" would be "as much as you can imagine."

You rated your sound tolerance problem as a "2." You said you would have rated it a zero except you are always concerned about sound causing your tinnitus to get worse. We discussed how this is definitely a concern for sounds that are so loud as to damage your ears, but for lower-level sounds this is not a problem for you.

Question 36. How much of a problem is *hearing*? "0" would be "no problem at all"; "10" would be "as much as you can imagine."

You rated your hearing problem as a "7."

WALKING YOU THROUGH THE TRT INITIAL INTERVIEW

Tinnitus Questionnaire

In chapter 2, I explained that, in addition to the TRT Initial Interview, it was also important to complete a traditional tinnitus questionnaire. We used the Tinnitus Functional Index (TFI) for that purpose. Your total (index) score on the TFI was 76, indicating that tinnitus severely affects your life. We also got scores for each of the eight subscales (domains—listed in chapter 2), which indicated that tinnitus affects all areas of your life, but mostly your emotional reactions, sleep, and ability to concentrate.

Summary of Your TRT Evaluation

If we look at your responses on the Tinnitus and Hearing Survey, your responses to questions 34, 35, and 36 from the TRT Initial Interview give us basically the same results. That is, you have a severe problem with tinnitus, a significant problem with hearing, and a very mild problem with sound tolerance. Your responses to the Tinnitus Functional Index were in agreement as to the severity of your tinnitus. Based on all your responses, you meet the criteria for TRT category 2. Treatment therefore needs to focus on your tinnitus, and hearing aids will be recommended for your hearing difficulties. The hearing aids will have a built-in sound generator, and we will use the sound generators as part of your treatment. Sound tolerance is a minimal issue for you, and the treatment for your tinnitus should also improve your mild sound tolerance problem. If the sound tolerance problem was severe, then we would focus on that first before treating the tinnitus.

PART 3

Walking You Through Treatment

CHAPTER 6

Sound Therapy for TRT

We completed your evaluation, which gave us both a good understanding of what should be most beneficial for your treatment. The bottom line is, your tinnitus is a significant problem *and* you have difficulties hearing. The hearing difficulties are the reason you will be treated as a category 2 rather than a category 1 patient (category 1 would be a tinnitus problem alone). Treatment for both categories 1 and 2 involves the full TRT counseling along with sound therapy using wearable ear-level devices. The only major difference in treatment for category 2 is the use of hearing aids with a built-in sound generator (combination instruments) rather than just wearable (ear-level) sound generators. In

> Treatment for both categories 1 and 2 involves the full TRT counseling along with sound therapy using wearable ear-level devices.

addition, the counseling for category 2 places an emphasis on hearing loss and how it may be involved in triggering and worsening tinnitus.[4]

Fitting Hearing Aids

Although technically you will be using combination instruments, we will refer to them as hearing aids.

You will wear a hearing aid in each ear. There are many types of hearing aids. You will be using the *behind-the-ear* type that hooks over the top of your ear and fits snugly between your ear and your skull. They are very small and will be hardly noticeable when you are wearing them.

Behind-the-ear hearing aids can use either a narrow tube for the sound to travel from the hearing aid to an earpiece in your ear canal, or a thin wire to connect to a receiver (like a tiny speaker) that is suspended in your ear canal (called a *receiver-in-canal* hearing aid). You will be using the receiver-in-canal style. An important benefit of this type of hearing aid is that it keeps your ear canal open. This is referred to as *open fit,* which is important to allow sound that surrounds you (ambient sound) to enter your ears in the normal fashion. Ambient sound combines with amplified sound from the hearing aid and the broadband noise from the sound generator.

We are fitting and adjusting the hearing aids in a reasonably quiet environment, which is the only time I will ask you to be in quiet (I will explain later why it is important to avoid silence). We do not do this fitting and adjusting, however, in a super-quiet testing booth, which would be an unrealistic environment with respect to your everyday use of the hearing aids. A little sound in the background makes the fitting more realistic. We are also covering all the important things you need to know about maintaining your hearing aids such as cleaning, batteries, and troubleshooting.

You mentioned that your tinnitus was slightly more bothersome in your right ear, so we will fit that ear first. We start by adjusting the output of the amplification portion prior to adjusting the level of the sound generator. The sound generator is adjusted to a level just below the *mixing point,* which I will explain next. The second device is then fit to your left ear. Again, we start by adjusting the amplification.

> The sound generator is adjusted to a level just below the mixing point...

The output of the left-side sound generator is then set to balance with the output of the right-side sound generator.

What Is the Mixing Point?

It has been difficult for many people to grasp the concept of the mixing point. It is a very important concept, so I need to explain it in detail. Because of its importance, every time you return to the clinic we will review how to adjust your sound generators to just below the mixing point.

The term *masking* refers to the use of sound to cover up (make inaudible) the sound of tinnitus. With TRT the word *suppression* is used instead because it is thought that suppression more correctly describes what takes place in the brain when sound makes tinnitus inaudible.[5,51] It is important to understand that a sound will cause one of three effects with respect to suppressing tinnitus: complete suppression, partial suppression, or no suppression. Complete suppression and no suppression are self-explanatory—with complete suppression, tinnitus cannot be heard; with no suppression, the tinnitus sound does not change.

> ...a sound will cause one of three effects with respect to suppressing tinnitus: complete suppression, partial suppression, or no suppression.

Partial suppression means the tinnitus sensation changes in some way when sound is presented. The change in the tinnitus sensation can be one or both of two possibilities.[52] First, the tinnitus does not seem as loud when exposed to the external sound. Second, the tinnitus sounds different in some way, which is typically due to some frequencies being enhanced and others reduced (like playing a chord on a piano and making some keys louder and others softer) and/or some frequencies (keys) being added and others omitted.

Tinnitus sounding different in some way is more technically referred to as a change in the *spectral characteristics* of tinnitus. It's also referred to as a change in the *quality* or the *timbre*—pronounced TAM-ber—of the tinnitus.

Here's what's important: The minimum level at which sound causes the spectral characteristics of tinnitus to change is what defines the mixing point. *Whether or not there is a reduction in the perceived loudness of the tinnitus is irrelevant.*

The minimum level at which sound causes the spectral characteristics of tinnitus to change is what defines the mixing point.

To summarize, the mixing point is an essential concept that relates to the adjustment of wearable sound generators. When adjusting the level of the sound, the lowest (*threshold*) level of the sound that is perceived to "mix," "blend," or "interfere" with the sound of the tinnitus defines the mixing point. As the sound generators are turned up (made louder) above the mixing point, the tinnitus can still be heard but it sounds different (or, more technically, it is perceived to have different spectral characteristics). This change in the sound of tinnitus is not related to its perceived loudness—any reduction in the perceived loudness is not relevant to the mixing point.

...any reduction in the perceived loudness is not relevant to the mixing point.

How to Adjust the Sound Generators

Now that you understand the concept of the mixing point, let's adjust your sound generators. You will note that we do not refer to them as noise generators because the word *noise* has negative connotations. The sound emitted from your sound generators needs to result in a totally positive experience.

> The sound generators are adjusted every time they are placed in your ears—*and at no other time.*

The sound generators are adjusted every time they are placed in your ears—*and at no other time.* The level of the sound is first adjusted to the mixing point and then reduced slightly so that it is perceived as being below the mixing point. The sound emitted from the devices should never cause any annoyance or discomfort, even if the sound never reaches the mixing point (which would be very uncommon). Any level of the sound below the mixing point—referred to as the *therapeutic range*—is effective to promote habituation.

> Any level of the sound below the mixing point—referred to as the *therapeutic range*—is effective to promote habituation.

Let's talk about the *therapeutic range* for sound from the sound generators and why it matters—on both the lower and upper ends of the range. The lowest end of the range is the softest level at which the sound can be heard—that level is the *threshold of audibility.* The sound should not be set very close to the threshold of audibility because of the potential for the sound to make the tinnitus louder. More technically, this concern is based on the principle of *stochastic resonance,* which means that sound that is close to the threshold of audibility can increase central auditory gain, which could *theoretically* increase the tinnitus loudness.[53] More simply, think of central auditory gain as a volume control in the brain.[41] A sound that is very close to threshold could turn up that volume control and potentially make the tinnitus louder.

The upper end of the therapeutic range is the mixing point. At and above the mixing point, the sound of the tinnitus (its spectrum, quality, or timbre) changes. This change must not occur during sound therapy because it will prevent you from habituating to your "usual" tinnitus. In addition, the sound from the sound generators must never cause any degree of annoyance. So the sound should never be so loud as to either change what the tinnitus sounds like or cause any annoyance.

After the first sound generator is adjusted to a comfortable level below the mixing point, the second sound generator is adjusted to match the perceived loudness of the first. I recall that you described your tinnitus as consisting of two sounds—a high-pitched squealing sound and a soft, low-pitched hum. The high-pitched sound is the dominant sound, and it is your most bothersome tinnitus, so that is the sound we will focus on. We can disregard the low-frequency hum—it may even be partially or completely suppressed in the process, which is acceptable.

The perceived loudness of the sound from the sound generator in the second ear should be the same as that in the first ear. If the sound causes annoyance or changes the tinnitus quality in either ear, then it should be decreased equally in both devices so that it is perceived as the same loudness in each ear.

Sound Generators: Points to Remember

> Sound generators are normally used for one to two years, or until at least three months after you feel they are no longer needed.

Sound generators are normally used for one to two years, or until at least three months after you feel they are no longer needed. Let's now review the important things to remember when using your sound generators:

1. Always adjust the sound to below the mixing point (within the therapeutic range) and below any level that would cause annoyance or discomfort after many hours of wearing the devices.
2. "Set and forget" means the sound generators should not be readjusted while they are being worn for any continuous period of time. Readjustment can cause you to pay attention to the devices and to your tinnitus, which would work against the efforts to promote habituation.
3. Wear the sound generators every day and as much as possible during the day. There is no need to wear them while sleeping.
4. Whether or not you are wearing your sound generators, always add comfortable sound to enrich your ambient sound environment all day, every day.
5. If there is any problem with the sound generators, promptly seek help from your clinician. Return them immediately if repair is needed.

CHAPTER 7

Background to the Neurophysiological Model

Before we start the TRT counseling, I need to explain a few things. The counseling you will receive is consistent with what was recommended by Dr. Pawel Jastreboff and Mr. Jonathan Hazell in their 2004 book, which they describe as "the definitive description and justification of the Jastreboff neurophysiological model of tinnitus."[4] They point out that "the principles on which it [the neurophysiological model] is based and its mechanisms are complex and their understanding requires knowledge from various areas of neuroscience. . . . the proper use of TRT only comes from a combination of a full understanding of the theory followed by significant practical experience of its use with patients."[(p. xii)] This quote might help explain why so many clinicians have difficulty learning and practicing TRT consistent with Jastreboff and Hazell's "definitive description and justification."

At this point you might be wondering, "If clinicians have difficulty understanding the TRT counseling, how can I possibly understand it?" Addressing that concern is the main reason I wrote this book. The counseling is as simplified and straightforward as I could make it. Knowing that you may need assistance finding a provider who thoroughly understands TRT, I have provided resources in chapter 10.

The counseling you are about to receive is the result of my carefully studying the description of TRT counseling in Jastreboff and Hazell's book—specifically pages 85 through 106.[4] I created exact wording (a script) that I suggested clinicians could use to deliver the TRT counseling to patients. The entire script was included in the book about TRT that I authored in 2007.[51] In addition, each scripted section corresponds directly to the companion book that I also authored, titled *Tinnitus Retraining Therapy: Patient Counseling Guide*.[10] The flip-chart format of the companion book helps to guide the counseling session and maintain consistency between visits and between clinicians. With each turn of the page, the clinician sees a bulleted list of key counseling points, and the patient sees mostly graphics that illustrate the information being taught.

The companion book contains 160 pages of counseling information, including 80 pages oriented to the clinician and 80 pages oriented to the patient.[10] An additional 14 pages guide the counseling for decreased sound tolerance (see appendix D). For the initial counseling visit, each page generally requires one minute or more to explain the contents. The entire visit may be completed within an hour and a half, although it is not unusual to require two hours or more. It is therefore often necessary for the counseling to be split up over two (or more) meetings.

The TRT neurophysiological model of tinnitus is typically shown as a graphic to support the counseling. The original book about TRT shows different detailed versions of the neurophysiological model.[4] Simplified versions are shown in the present book. The model shows how different areas of the brain that we will be discussing are connected. The important point is that these areas *are* connected, and some of those connections need to be broken, or at least modified, for habituation to occur. A basic version of the neurophysiological model as it pertains to the processing of external sound is provided in Figure 7-1.

TRT counseling can be described as *educational sessions to create a new frame of reference for thinking about your tinnitus.*[8] The objectives of the counseling are to *demystify* and *reclassify* the tinnitus neural signal that is stored in your memory. It will also be important to understand the rationale and importance of maintaining an enriched environment of non-annoying sounds to maximize treatment effects.

> The objectives of the counseling are to *demystify* and *reclassify* the tinnitus neural signal that is stored in your memory.

More importantly, the counseling is based on the neurophysiological model of tinnitus (see Figure 7-2), which shows brain areas that are activated when tinnitus is bothersome.[4] And *most* importantly, the counseling provides plenty of opportunity for you to ask questions. So in that sense, the counseling is bidirectional.

The counseling covers six major topics: (1) overview of the auditory system, (2) hearing and the brain, (3) rules of perception, (4) limitation of attention, (5) plasticity of the brain, and (6) the neurophysiological model of tinnitus.

7-1. Basis for the Neurophysiological Model. This illustration shows how different brain areas can be activated when sound enters the ears. An external sound (lower left in the figure) activates the cochlea and auditory subconscious (solid lines). If there is awareness of the sound, then the auditory cortex is also activated (dashed line). A sound that carries emotional significance would also activate the limbic system and autonomic nervous system (dashed lines). (Figure adapted from Jastreboff and Hazell, 2004[4])

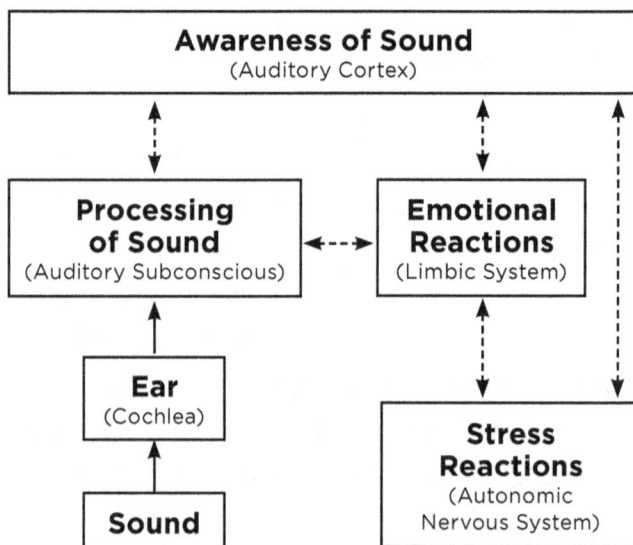

Another topic is provided for treatment of decreased sound tolerance, which is covered in appendix D.

The first five topics are background information that will help you understand the neurophysiological model (Figs. 7-1 and 7-2). The background information is covered in this chapter. In the next chapter, I will spend considerable time explaining the neurophysiological model. This will comprise a substantial amount of new and fairly technical information that would be difficult for anyone to fully

7-2. The Neurophysiological Model of Tinnitus. Like sound, tinnitus can activate different areas of the brain. Tinnitus that is bothersome activates the auditory cortex, the limbic system, and the autonomic nervous system. All brain areas that are activated by bothersome tinnitus are shown by the solid lines. (Figure adapted from Jastreboff and Hazell, 2004[4])

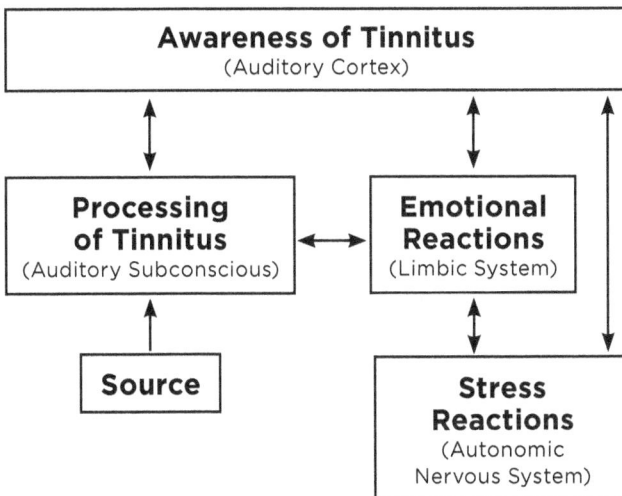

Awareness of Tinnitus
(Auditory Cortex)

Processing of Tinnitus
(Auditory Subconscious)

Emotional Reactions
(Limbic System)

Source

Stress Reactions
(Autonomic Nervous System)

comprehend in one sitting. The main objective is that you understand the essence of each major concept. We will only cover as much material as you can comfortably understand. When you reach a saturation point, we'll stop and pick up later where we left off.

Topic 1: Overview of the Auditory System

Many theories have been proposed about what causes tinnitus.[54,55] In spite of all the research that has been done, no one yet has all the answers. A good place to start on the path to understanding tinnitus is to understand how our hearing system works. Understanding the hearing system can help to demystify tinnitus—it's like opening a mysterious black box and discovering what's inside.

We will now describe the hearing system, from the outer ear all the way to the top of the brain. Understanding how the hearing system works will help you to better understand your test results and establish a foundation for the upcoming counseling that will focus on tinnitus.

Sound Waves

Our *acoustic environment* is the three-dimensional landscape of ambient sounds that we are surrounded by almost every waking minute. A physical event is responsible for every sound by generating *sound waves*. (Here's the answer to the question, "When a tree falls in the forest, does it make a sound?" The falling tree generates sound waves regardless of whether anyone is there to process the sound waves that would enable the sound to be perceived.) Sound waves emanate from the physical event in all directions—like an expanding balloon. They contain energy and cause objects to vibrate—objects like our eardrums. The primary factor distinguishing tinnitus from other sounds is that *tinnitus is not associated with a sound wave.*

> The primary factor distinguishing tinnitus from other sounds is that *tinnitus is not associated with a sound wave.*

The Hearing System

For simplicity, the hearing system consists of two major divisions: the *ear* and the *auditory nervous system.* Portions of the ear work like a microphone by vibrating when struck by sound waves and converting the vibrations to a different form of energy. The auditory nervous system works like a computer to process and interpret the signals coming from the ear. The ear and the auditory nervous system are connected by the *auditory nerve,* which we can think of as a cable that connects the microphone and the computer.

The Ear (Fig. 7-3)

Most of the ear is embedded in the skull on the side of the head. The ear's job is to convert the physical vibrations caused by sound waves into nerve impulses—like a microphone converts sound waves into electrical signals. The ear consists of the outer ear, middle ear, and inner ear.

7-3. Anatomy of the Ear. Sound enters the ear canal and vibrates the eardrum. The vibrations are transmitted to the cochlea via the middle ear bones (hammer, anvil, and stirrup). Hair cells in the cochlea convert the vibrations to neural signals that are sent into the brain via the auditory nerve. (Illustration created by Lynn H. Kitagawa, MFA)

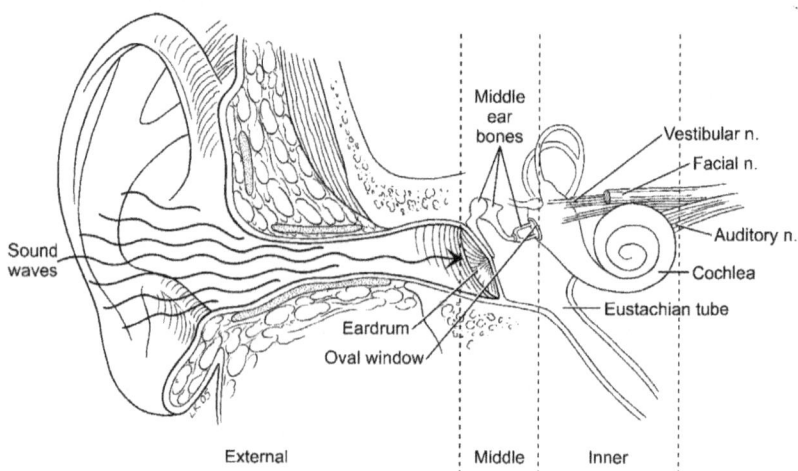

The *outer ear* is the part of the ear that is seen on the side of the head, and it includes the ear canal. The outer ear channels sound waves to the eardrum.

The *middle ear* is like a tiny room that is dedicated to getting sound vibrations from the outer ear to the inner ear. (It accomplishes this very efficiently by what is known as *impedance matching*.) The middle ear includes the eardrum and the *ossicles* (the three middle ear bones: malleus, incus, and stapes—often referred as the hammer, anvil, and stirrup). Sound waves strike the eardrum and travel through the ossicles to the inner ear. The ossicles are connected to tiny muscles that stiffen the bones when needed to reduce the intensity of sound entering the inner ear. That stiffening provides some level of protection from loud sounds.

The *inner ear* is a bony structure that includes the *cochlea*. The cochlea is shaped like a snail shell and is about the size of the tip of your little finger. The cochlea is filled with fluid; sound vibrations cause movement in the fluid, which activates special sensory cells called *hair cells*.

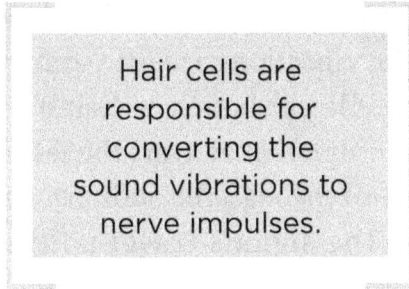

> Hair cells are responsible for converting the sound vibrations to nerve impulses.

Hair cells are responsible for converting the sound vibrations to nerve impulses.

Auditory Nerve: The "Cable"

The hair cells send their signals through the auditory nerve to the brain stem (Fig. 7-3). Think of the auditory nerve as a very short cable that contains thousands of individual wires. Each "wire" is a nerve fiber.

Auditory Nervous System: The "Computer"

Signals from the auditory nerve enter the brain stem and are then relayed through several brain centers up to the outermost layer of the brain (the *auditory cortex*), where hearing actually occurs. These brain centers are called *nuclei*, which are clusters of neurons. Each cluster has a dedicated role in the processing of auditory information.

Topic 2: Hearing and the Brain

Let's review what we've covered so far. Sound waves travel through the ear canal and cause the eardrum to vibrate. The vibrations are transmitted to the cochlea via the three middle ear bones (ossicles). In the cochlea, hair cells (the microphone) convert the vibrations to nerve signals, which travel through the auditory nerve (the cable) into the brain. As the signals travel up through the auditory nervous system (the computer), they undergo complex processing by brain centers. Conscious perception of sound in the auditory cortex is the result of this sequence of activity.

With that overview of how the hearing system works, we will now go into greater detail to describe *how* sound waves are converted to nerve impulses and then processed by the auditory nervous system.

Organ of Corti

The organ of Corti is an elaborate strip of membrane contained within the cochlea. The hair cells that convert sound vibrations into nerve impulses are embedded in the organ of Corti.

The Piano Keyboard in the Cochlea

We can think of the organ of Corti as a piano keyboard of sorts (Fig. 7-4). The hair cells are like keys on the piano and are *tuned* to be responsive to certain frequencies. And, just like a piano, lower frequencies are on one end of the organ of Corti, and they gradually become higher pitched at the other end.

7-4. Surface View of Hair Cells in the Organ of Corti. There is one row of inner hair cells and three rows of outer hair cells. The piano keyboard represents how the hair cells are laid out, with low frequencies on one end progressing to high frequencies on the other. On the right is an artist's rendition of how the different frequencies correspond to different regions of the cochlea. (Scanning electron photomicrograph courtesy of David J. Lim, MD, House Ear Institute; illustrations created by Lynn H. Kitagawa, MFA)

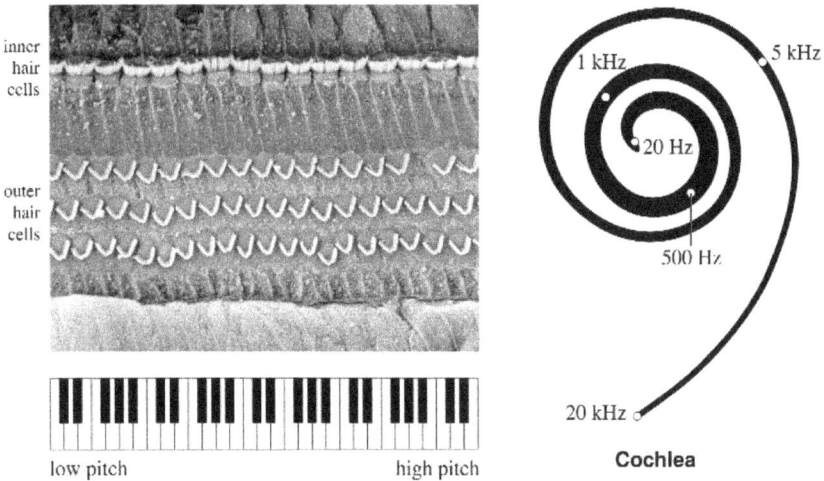

inner hair cells

outer hair cells

low pitch   high pitch

1 kHz   5 kHz

20 Hz

500 Hz

20 kHz

Cochlea

Hair Cells

Hair cells activate auditory neural signals that travel into the brain stem. There are about 16,000 hair cells contained within each cochlea. The hair cells are spaced evenly along the organ of Corti, with one row of inner hair cells next to three rows of outer hair cells (Fig. 7-4).

The Amplifier in the Cochlea

What's the difference between inner hair cells and outer hair cells? They have different roles. Inner hair cells respond to vibrations and send neural signals into the brain. Inner hair cells cannot, however, detect vibrations caused by softer sounds. That is the job of the outer hair cells—they are sensitive to softer sounds and *amplify* them so that they can be detected by the inner hair cells. (Outer hair cells have been referred to as the "amplifier in the cochlea.")

Damage to Hair Cells

All hair cells—outer or inner—can be damaged or destroyed (Fig. 7-5). Outer hair cells are more easily damaged than inner hair cells. The damage can be temporary or permanent. For example, temporary damage can be caused by exposure to loud noise, with recovery taking place after a few days or so. With repeated exposure (or if the noise is extremely loud), the damage can become permanent without any possibility of recovery.

7-5. Surface View of Normal and Damaged Hair Cells. Normal (undamaged) hair cells are on the left. A typical pattern of hair cell damage (damaged outer hair cells and intact inner hair cells) is shown on the right. (Scanning electron photomicrographs courtesy of David J. Lim, MD, House Ear Institute)

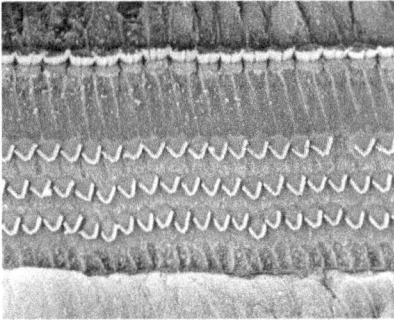

Normal hair cells

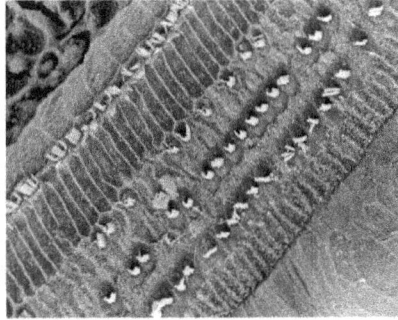

Damaged hair cells

Loss of Hair Cells and Normal Hearing

If the outer hair cell loss is fairly evenly distributed along the organ of Corti, up to 30% of the cells can be destroyed and a person's hearing sensitivity will remain mostly intact (Fig. 7-5). When hearing thresholds are tested, the audiogram will look normal. Hair cells are able to compensate for this amount of loss before the ability to hear is affected noticeably.

Everyone loses outer hair cells at the rate of about one-half percent per year from the moment of birth.

Everyone loses outer hair cells at the rate of about one-half percent per year from the moment of birth. At that rate, hearing loss would not begin to be noticeable until age 60 or so. That, of course, assumes that nothing has accelerated the damage, such as loud noise, drugs that are *ototoxic,* viral infections, or autoimmune or other medical disorders. Regardless of whether hair cell loss is natural due to aging or caused by something else, the damage tends to start in higher-frequency regions of the cochlea, with progression to lower-frequency regions over time.

Hair Cell Loss: Outer versus Inner

Here's something really interesting. There are three times as many outer hair cells as inner hair cells (Fig. 7-4). However, 95% of auditory nerve fibers are connected to inner hair cells—only 5% are connected to outer hair cells. Complete loss of outer hair cells would result in about a 50 decibel (dB) loss of hearing sensitivity across all frequencies (the audiogram would show a *flat* 50 dB hearing loss). Complete loss of inner hair cells—regardless of whether outer hair cells remain intact—would result in *total* hearing loss. Usually there are regions along the organ of Corti that have more damage than other regions (similar to male pattern baldness). A region with complete loss of inner hair cells would result in a complete loss of hearing *in the corresponding frequency range.*

Otoacoustic Emissions

We just mentioned that there are usually regions along the organ of Corti that have more damage than other regions.

These patches of damage may not result in any noticeable loss of hearing because healthy cells that are adjacent to the damaged region compensate for the missing cells. It is possible to detect these regions with testing for *distortion-product otoacoustic emissions* (DPOAE; see appendix C). DPOAE is one specific way to detect otoacoustic emissions, which are "echoes" in the ear canal. These echoes are caused by outer hair cells literally lengthening and shortening in response to vibrations in the cochlear fluid. This lengthening and shortening is how outer hair cells amplify softer sounds so that they can be detected by the less-sensitive inner hair cells.

Discordant Damage or Dysfunction

According to Dr. Jastreboff, these regions of damage to outer hair cells may play a role in the onset and maintenance of tinnitus. The damaged regions are adjacent to inner hair cells that are intact or much less damaged (Fig. 7-5). The net effect is that areas of *discordant damage or dysfunction* could be the source of tinnitus, even if the damage is minor and hearing is normal.[55]

> ...regions of damage to outer hair cells may play a role in the onset and maintenance of tinnitus.

Discordant Damage/Dysfunction Theory

Here's how discordant damage or dysfunction of hair cells might explain tinnitus. We've discussed how nerve fibers from both the outer and inner hair cells enter the brain stem and start getting processed by different brain centers. The first brain center that does the processing is the *cochlear nucleus.*

Outer and inner hair cells from the same region of the cochlea activate fibers in the auditory nerve that connect to the same region of the cochlear nucleus. In other words, hair cell activity in one region of the cochlea activates a corresponding region in the cochlear nucleus. It's like there is a piano keyboard in the cochlea, and the same layout of piano keys is preserved in the cochlear nucleus and all the way up the auditory nervous system (this configuration is technically referred to as *tonotopic organization*).

Here's what Dr. Jastreboff theorizes: Our entire nervous system involves combinations of excitation and inhibition. Inhibition keeps the excitation in check. Normally, auditory nerve fibers from the same region in the cochlea balance each other to maintain normal nerve activity being sent further up the auditory pathways. This balance is due to fibers from outer hair cells inhibiting the excitatory output of fibers from inner hair cells.[56,57] Discordant damage or dysfunction (regions of outer hair cells missing and inner hair cells intact) results in fibers from the inner hair cells sending normal excitatory signals, *but without the inhibition coming from the corresponding region of outer hair cells.* This imbalance has been shown to cause abnormal bursting activity in the *dorsal* portion of the cochlear nucleus.[58] This bursting activity becomes amplified and is then perceived as tinnitus. That's the theory.

Neural Networks

The auditory nervous system begins with the hair cells in the cochlea and includes all of the associated pathways that connect with the auditory cortex. These pathways are extremely complex and consist of bundles of interconnected nerve cells, called *neural networks*, that process the incoming auditory signals. This processing includes recognizing patterns of neural activity and blocking signals that are unimportant or irrelevant to the person's needs.

Enhancement and Suppression of Neural Activity

Neurons in the brain have extensive connections with each other. There are two basic features of connections between individual neurons: (1) The sending neuron causes either excitation (enhancement) or inhibition (suppression) of activity in the receiving neuron. (2) These connections are continually changing such that the activity of receiving neurons is either increased or decreased. Networks of neurons (neural networks) are capable of processing many different signals simultaneously. Some of these signals are enhanced and some are suppressed.

Auditory Gain

The auditory nervous system has *gain control*, kind of like the volume knob on a radio in older cars. The *level of auditory gain* (where the volume knob is set) determines how much

> The auditory nervous system has *gain control*, kind of like the volume knob on a radio in older cars.

environmental sounds are amplified, or enhanced, in the auditory nervous system.

The level of auditory gain is always self-adjusting to adapt to how much sound is entering the ear canals. If the sound level *decreases*, auditory gain increases (that is, softer sounds result in "turning up the volume"). If the sound level *increases*, auditory gain decreases (that is, louder sounds result in "turning down the volume"). Auditory gain is partially controlled by the outer hair cells, which amplify softer sounds (as we discussed), and partially by neural networks that adjust to different levels of sound.

The Heller and Bergman Experiment

This experiment was reported over 70 years ago but is still very relevant to understanding tinnitus.[59] During the experiment, people *who did not have tinnitus* were seated with pencil and paper in a quiet sound booth and instructed to write down "any sounds they might hear." Within five minutes of being seated with the door closed, 94% of these 80 individuals reported whistling, pulsing, and buzzing sounds. The sounds they wrote down were identical

> ...under certain circumstances, perceiving tinnitus is an inherent property of the auditory nervous system.

to the types of sounds that would be described by people with tinnitus.

This experiment clearly demonstrated that, under certain circumstances, perceiving tinnitus is an inherent property of the auditory nervous system. The perception of tinnitus is therefore not necessarily the result of some pathological process.

Why Is the Heller and Bergman Experiment Important?

All nerve fibers send impulses (like sending a signal through a wire) spontaneously and randomly. These impulses occur without any triggering event. For neurons in the auditory nervous system, these random impulses occur 50 to 100 times every second *when there is no sound*. When there *is* sound, the random activity becomes more patterned and the brain recognizes different patterns as different sounds (the brain really does work like a computer). The patterned activity starts in the cochlea and then travels through the auditory nerve and up the auditory pathways to the auditory cortex, where the sound is consciously perceived.

The auditory nervous system recognizes different patterns of neural activity as different sounds. Any background random activity is automatically filtered out and therefore not consciously perceived as sound.

We discussed the concept of auditory gain, which is useful to help explain the significance of the Heller and Bergman experiment. Recall that if the level (loudness) of sound *decreases*, auditory gain increases (softer sounds result in "turning up the volume"). When a person is in a very quiet environment (such as a sound booth), auditory gain may increase to the point that the brain interprets the random activity as sound—hence, tinnitus. The takeaway message is that *almost everyone has tinnitus if it is quiet enough*. It is therefore possible that, for some people, tinnitus is associated with increased auditory gain.

> ...*almost everyone has tinnitus if it is quiet enough.*

Topic 3: Rules of Perception

When you have your hearing evaluated, one of the main objectives is to measure your hearing thresholds (the softest sounds you can hear). This testing is done under controlled conditions—including a super-quiet sound booth. These controlled conditions, however, do not represent how we hear in everyday surroundings. Our hearing is often challenged by having to pick out sounds (usually speech) that are embedded in a background of sound (for example, carrying on a conversation in a noisy restaurant). We are able to identify individual sounds in a complex mix of sounds because our neural networks are trained, through repeated exposure to sounds, to recognize the patterns of neural activity produced by the sounds.

Some sounds carry special meaning, such as our name. The neural networks in our auditory system become fine-tuned to detect such sounds. This explains why we notice our name being spoken in a noisy environment, even if we are engaged in a separate conversation. This phenomenon, known as *the cocktail party effect*, can also happen with tinnitus. The ongoing presence of tinnitus can train neural networks to detect the tinnitus neural signal with great precision. If the tinnitus signal carries special meaning because of past associations, the signal will be easily detected by the brain, even in the midst of other auditory signals.

> If the tinnitus signal carries special meaning because of past associations, the signal will be easily detected by the brain, even in the midst of other auditory signals.

Perception of Signal Strength

Anything we see or hear is the result of sensory stimuli, which we will refer to as *signals*. One of the qualities of any signal is its strength—its brightness to the eyes or its loudness to the ears. Our perception of signal strength does not depend just on the absolute physical intensity of a signal. Rather, our perception of signal strength depends mainly upon its *relative* strength compared to surrounding signals. For example, we would perceive a candle flame in a dark room as bright and impossible to ignore (Fig 7-6). With the lights turned on, however, the candle flame is barely

> ...our perception of signal strength depends mainly upon its *relative* strength compared to surrounding signals.

noticeable. When the lights were turned on, the *same* candle flame changed from being perceived as a strong signal to being perceived as a weak signal.

7-6. Candle as an Example of Relative Signal Strength. The candle is the same in the dark room (A) and the lighted room (B), but it is *less noticeable* in the lighted room because of the reduced contrast. (Illustrations created by Lynn H. Kitagawa, MFA)

A

B

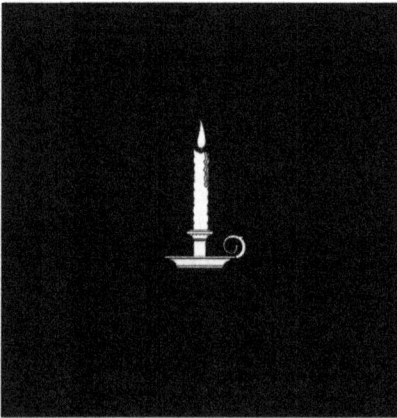
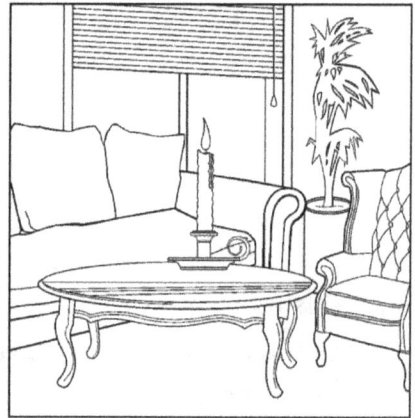

As another example, let's say you're conversing with a friend while working outside on a quiet sunny day. Suddenly a lawnmower is running next door, and you have to practically yell to hear each other. When the lawnmower is turned off, you again talk at a normal level. The strength of your voices was relative to the surrounding (ambient) sound.

Perception of Tinnitus Strength

Just like your voices seemed louder when the lawnmower was turned off, your tinnitus seems to get louder when you move to a quiet environment (Fig. 7-7). For example, when you climb into bed after a busy day, all or most of the background sound suddenly stops. *The silence causes your tinnitus to seem louder.* For this reason, it is important to avoid silence. Always maintain some background sound to reduce the *perceived* loudness of your tinnitus and decrease the relative strength of the tinnitus neural signal.

7-7. Tinnitus Seems Louder in Quiet. As for the candle in Figure 7-6, the word *tinnitus* is the same in both A and B, but it is less noticeable in B because of the reduced contrast. This exemplifies how tinnitus seems louder in a quiet background and not as loud when there is a background of sound. (Illustrations created by Lynn H. Kitagawa, MFA)

A

B

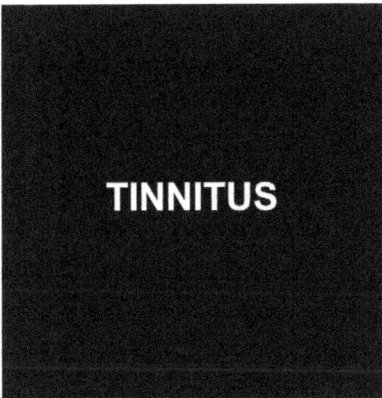
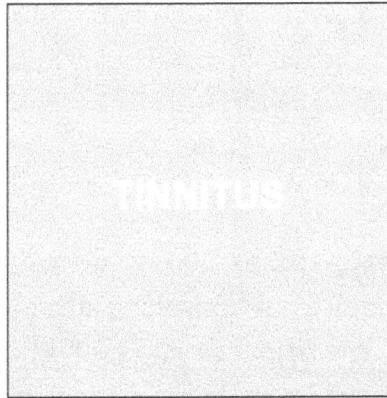

Topic 4: Limitation of Attention

The brain is capable of performing any number of complex tasks. Some tasks require our full attention, such as reading a book or writing a letter. We cannot do two of these kinds of tasks simultaneously. It has to be one or the other.

Sensory Overload

Sensory stimuli (sights and sounds) usually flood our eyes and ears, but they don't normally cause *sensory overload*. With respect to the auditory system, all of the sounds we are exposed to activate the hair cells in the cochlea, and the corresponding vibrations are converted to neural signals that are sent into the brain for processing—this can be a flood of incoming auditory information. How does the brain distinguish and separate all these signals and determine what's most important? Several strategies are used by the brain to ensure that only those signals that are most important at a given moment reach our awareness. Let's discuss three strategies the brain uses to manage sensory overload.

Managing Sensory Overload: (1) Automated Responses

Many things that we do are mostly automatic—they do not require our conscious attention. This is explainable because of *conditioned reflexes*. Walking, running, climbing stairs, and riding a bike all involve routine, predictable responses that we learn naturally while growing up. Playing a musical instrument becomes almost automatic with enough practice. Driving a car requires continuous processing of a huge amount of complex information, but we can safely drive while carrying on a conversation (provided we don't take our eyes off the road!). Anything we do that is automatic frees up the brain to pay conscious attention to something else.

> Anything we do that is automatic frees up the brain to pay conscious attention to something else.

Managing Sensory Overload: (2) Classification of Signals

Imagine cleaning out a room and deciding what to keep and what not to keep. Some things are considered important and others unimportant. The brain does the same thing with sensory information (signals). It subconsciously classifies each incoming signal as important or unimportant.

An important signal causes some consequence—either positive (reward) or negative (punishment). Whether reward or punishment, the consequence reinforces the signal's importance and the need to pay attention to it. When a signal is classified as important, it is not blocked from reaching conscious attention and serves as an alert that some action may need to be taken.

A signal is classified as unimportant if it is experienced repeatedly and without consequences (without reinforcement). An unimportant signal is a *neutral* signal—it is normally blocked from reaching conscious attention and does not evoke any reactions. Unimportant signals therefore do not normally interfere with our ability to pay attention to important signals.

Managing Sensory Overload: (3) Prioritization of Signals

Let's go back to our example of cleaning out a room. We might want to assign numbers to each item to indicate its importance relative to other items, for example on a scale of 0 to 10. This would help us to decide which items are essential (labeled a "10"), which are nonessential (labeled a "0"), and which are somewhere in between (labeled between 1 and 9). In effect we are ranking each item in terms of its *priority*.

The brain automatically ranks signals *according to their relative priority*. Signals ranked as a 10 on the priority scale require immediate attention, and others receive attention in order of decreasing priority. For example, a signal that induces fear or is perceived as threatening will cause immediate action.

> The brain automatically ranks signals *according to their relative priority.*

Let's say you're walking in the woods, and you hear the sound of an approaching tiger. That sound will completely dominate your attention until you know you are out of danger. This response is automatic and beyond your control. Now imagine attending a counseling session. A tiger is lying in the corner, and the counselor assures you the tiger is friendly. Regardless of the counselor's assurance, the tiger completely draws your attention away from the conversation. Tinnitus that is *perceived* as threatening can cause the same type of reaction.

Topic 5: Plasticity of the Brain

The brain undergoes continuous change—this basic characteristic is referred to as *plasticity.* Plastic changes occur in the synapses, which are the connections between neurons. The changes include new connections between neurons and modifications in the strength of existing connections. When we acquire new memories, either for conscious information or for conditioned reflexes, they are the result of changes in synapses.

> The brain undergoes continuous change—this basic characteristic is referred to as *plasticity.*

A basic principle of learning is that relearning something takes longer than if nothing was learned to begin with. For example, if we want to learn to properly swing a golf club, we will learn it more quickly if we had never swung a club than if we already play golf with a faulty swing.

> ...relearning something takes longer than if nothing was learned to begin with.

Retraining of Conditioned Reflexes

Conditioned reflexes are a form of learning. Once learned, a conditioned reflex can be relearned (or *retrained*). Tinnitus

Retraining Therapy refers to *retraining conditioned reflexes*. Retraining conditioned reflexes, however, requires that certain exercises are performed over a period of time. Retraining cannot occur just by using thought (cognitive) processes.

Tinnitus Retraining Therapy refers to *retraining conditioned reflexes.*

Tinnitus that is *not bothersome* is a manifestation of heightened spontaneous activity of neurons in the auditory nervous system—*only* in the auditory nervous system. When tinnitus is *bothersome,* the tinnitus neural signal is linked to areas of the brain responsible for feelings of annoyance and stress. This link is the conditioned reflex that needs to be retrained using proper exercises. More specifically, the reflex needs to be *extinguished.* Just like the faulty golf swing, bothersome tinnitus means a strong emotional association has been learned. The relearning process normally requires months or even a year or more.

Nonauditory Systems Activated by Tinnitus

The brain contains many different systems—each with a specific function. There is also interaction between systems. The auditory nervous system is dedicated to processing auditory information. The tinnitus neural signal is contained in the auditory nervous system, but if it is bothersome, the *limbic system* and the *autonomic nervous system* are activated by the tinnitus signal (Fig. 7-2).

Limbic System

The brain's limbic system is responsible for emotions. The limbic system and the auditory nervous system are connected, which is how sounds can evoke emotional responses when they are associated with certain memories (Fig. 7-1). Typical examples of sounds that can cause emotional reactions are certain pieces of music, a crying baby, or a particular person's voice. *If a sound does not evoke activity in the limbic system, the sound will be spontaneously and automatically habituated.*

> If a sound does not evoke activity in the limbic system, the sound will be spontaneously and automatically habituated.

Autonomic Nervous System

The autonomic nervous system is responsible for controlling basic bodily functions such as breathing, body temperature, heartbeat, blood pressure, sweating, and many others. All of these functions are automatic and normally beyond our ability to control. The bodily functions can, however, be modified by exercising or relaxing. Also, methods such as biofeedback and hypnosis attempt to modify these automatic functions by providing some degree of control over the autonomic nervous system.

Fight-or-Flight Response

The autonomic nervous system has a *sympathetic* part and a *parasympathetic* part (Table 7-1). Sensing danger or being fearful causes the sympathetic part of the autonomic nervous system to become strongly activated. This activation causes changes in the body that prepare it for *fight-or-flight*. These changes include adrenaline release into the bloodstream, increased heart rate, increased rate of breathing, increased muscle tension, and shutdown of digestive functions. The fight-or-flight reaction is so strong that it cannot be sustained for very long.

In contrast, if a stimulus has positive associations—for example, pleasant music—the parasympathetic part of the autonomic nervous system is activated. Parasympathetic activation is always working to counteract sympathetic activation. The parasympathetic system has been referred to as the *rest-and-digest* system.

> Parasympathetic activation is always working to counteract sympathetic activation.

Table 7-1. Effects of the Autonomic Nervous System. How body organs are affected by the two divisions of the autonomic nervous system: the parasympathetic and sympathetic nervous systems.

	Parasympathetic Nervous System	Sympathetic Nervous System
Overall Effect on the Body	Body at rest ("rest-and-digest")	Body prepared for emergency response ("fight-or-flight")
Heart	Beats normally	Beats faster
Muscles	Normal blood flow to skeletal muscles	Increased blood flow to skeletal muscles
Lungs	Airways constricted for relaxed breathing	Airways opened to increase oxygen
Digestion	Normal digestion	Digestive function slowed or stopped
Eyes	Normal pupil opening	Pupils dilated

Chronic Stress

Fear or danger activates the autonomic nervous system. When there is a need for physical or mental action, the sympathetic part of the autonomic nervous system is triggered (Table 7-1). This is a completely normal function that ensures that we do the things necessary for optimizing our lives and ultimately, for our survival.

The normal activation of the sympathetic part of the autonomic nervous system can become abnormal if the activation is *sustained*. Sustained activation may not be strong enough to induce the fight-or-flight response, but it can result in *chronic stress*. Chronic stress can have unhealthy consequences such as sleep deprivation, exhaustion, decreased energy, anxiety, and trouble concentrating. Experiencing chronic stress can greatly impact a person's quality of life.

Tinnitus and Stress

Back to tinnitus. If the tinnitus neural signal acquires associations with negative memories, the signal may be monitored both by conscious awareness of it and by subconscious processes. Such continual monitoring can cause sustained activation of the sympathetic part of the autonomic nervous system (Table 7-1), resulting in chronic stress. The level of sustained activation is dependent on the strength of negative associations acquired by the tinnitus.

CHAPTER 8

Explaining the Neurophysiological Model

We have so far covered a lot of information—some of it quite technical. Everything to this point is considered background information to help you understand the neuro-physiological model of tinnitus.

To make sure there is no confusion, *physiological* refers to functioning of systems and organs in the body. *Neuro-physiological* refers specifically to functioning of nervous systems in the body. The *neurophysiological model of tinnitus* describes how brain systems are functionally involved when a person has tinnitus. Importantly, TRT is not based on some sort of *psychological* model.

Let's review: We focused on three major areas of the brain—the auditory nervous system, the limbic system, and the autonomic nervous system. The auditory nervous system processes neural signals that enter the brain through the auditory nerve. If a sound evokes any type of emotional reaction, then it activates the limbic system. If the sound activating the limbic system has negative associations, then it causes activity in the sympathetic part of the autonomic nervous system. If the sympathetic activity is extreme, many changes take place in the body to prepare it for fight-or-flight. If the sympathetic activity is more moderate, but sustained over time, the same reactions will occur but to a lesser degree—resulting in chronic stress (the nervous system is on "high alert").

Conditioned Reflexes

> The tinnitus signal all by itself is harmless.

The tinnitus signal all by itself is harmless. That bears repeating—*the tinnitus signal all by itself is harmless.* Tinnitus is a problem only if it is linked to the limbic and autonomic nervous systems, which are largely controlled by conditioned reflexes.

We've discussed how conditioned reflexes can be caused by tinnitus. Reflexes triggered by tinnitus, however, are inappropriate because *they cause reactions to a harmless stimulus.* These reactions can range from mild to severe depending on the

> Reflexes triggered by tinnitus, however, are inappropriate because they cause reactions to a harmless stimulus.

degree of activation of the autonomic nervous system. The more it is activated, the more the tinnitus increases in severity.

No-Problem Tinnitus

It is estimated that 10 to 15% of all adults experience persistent tinnitus.[60] For about 80% of those people with tinnitus, it does not carry any special meaning and habituation takes place naturally and spontaneously. The brain learns that the tinnitus signal is insignificant, like the sound of a new refrigerator. When that happens, the tinnitus is classified by the brain as an unimportant signal. The signal is normally blocked (filtered out) from activating the limbic and autonomic nervous systems and from reaching conscious awareness. The tinnitus signal may be present all the time, but the person is usually not aware of it.

Problem Tinnitus

For the other 20% or so of people with persistent tinnitus, it's a different story.[14] Their tinnitus acquires special meaning because it is associated with something negative. The tinnitus signal is therefore classified by the brain as important.

Often, a negative connotation occurs when tinnitus is first experienced together with or shortly after an unpleasant or traumatic event.[61,62] The event triggers anxiety and annoyance, and these emotions become linked to the tinnitus. From the perspective of the neurophysiological model, an active connection is established between the auditory

> This connection causes increased activity in the limbic and autonomic nervous systems, *which is the underlying reason why tinnitus is bothersome.*

nervous system, which contains the tinnitus neural signal, and the limbic and autonomic nervous systems (Fig. 7-2). This connection causes increased activity in the limbic and autonomic nervous systems, *which is the underlying reason why tinnitus is bothersome.*

The Vicious Circle

When people first become aware of their tinnitus, initial curiosity may escalate into feelings of annoyance and anxiety. Such feelings reveal that the limbic system has been activated and the tinnitus signal has taken on the meaning of a threatening stimulus. Any neural signal that is recognized as threatening receives special attention from neural networks that become highly tuned to monitor the signal. Monitoring the signal means paying more conscious attention to the signal, which increases activation of the limbic and autonomic nervous systems. This activation, in turn, further enhances awareness of the signal. And so on—a vicious circle becomes established between awareness of the tinnitus and annoyance caused by the tinnitus.

> ...a vicious circle becomes established between awareness of the tinnitus and annoyance caused by the tinnitus.

Effects of Tinnitus

The repeating cycle (vicious circle) of awareness → reactions → awareness creates a high level of activation of the sympathetic part of the autonomic nervous system and ultimately chronic stress (Table 7-1). As we've already discussed, chronic stress can cause many harmful effects in the body.

Sleep Deprivation

Most people with bothersome tinnitus experience enhanced perception of their tinnitus when trying to sleep because of the quiet environment. Tinnitus can interfere with falling asleep, but it is more often reported to interfere with *maintaining* sleep.[4]

If tinnitus interferes with sleep night after night, sleep deprivation can become the main concern. When that occurs, it may be difficult to distinguish between effects caused by the tinnitus and those caused by the sleep deprivation. Those effects include exhaustion, perceptual distortions, illogical thinking, irritability, and difficulty performing tasks that require concentration.[63] Sleep deprivation can also lead to making irrational associations, which can lead to further annoyance due to the tinnitus.

Medications for Sleep

It is not uncommon for people with bothersome tinnitus to use prescription medications as an aid to sleeping. Medications may assist in prolonging a night's sleep, but they also may inhibit REM (rapid eye movement) sleep. The REM stage of sleep normally occurs four to five times a night and is critical for regulating our emotions and enabling mental concentration.

Some medications directly affect the limbic system, and they may be viewed as the only way to get relief from the effects of tinnitus. Using medications for this purpose may be necessary for short-term relief, but their long-term use can keep the vicious circle of tinnitus awareness and reactions from being broken. There is also the concern for negative side effects and becoming dependent on drugs just to carry on normal everyday activities. Importantly, some medications and interactions between medications can actually cause tinnitus or worsen existing tinnitus.

Tinnitus Loudness and Tinnitus Severity

A tinnitus evaluation often includes assessing its perceived loudness and pitch, which is typically done with the same audiometer that is used to measure hearing thresholds (appendix C). The result is a match between a tone's loudness and the loudness of the tinnitus (a *loudness match*) and a match between a tone's frequency and the pitch of the tinnitus (a *pitch match*). After the testing is complete you might be told something like, "Your tinnitus was matched to a 6000-hertz (Hz) tone at 10 decibels (dB) above your hearing threshold at the same frequency."

Obtaining loudness and pitch matches can be helpful if they give you assurance that the phantom sound in your head has been validated and quantified. Otherwise, it is well known that *these measures are not related to the degree of distress caused by the tinnitus.*[36] Often the measures seem to contradict each other. For example, a person may have a small loudness match but be very distressed by the tinnitus. Or a person may have a large loudness match but not be bothered at all by the tinnitus. These kinds of results are explainable by the neurophysiological model. The loudness and pitch of tinnitus reflect activity in the auditory nervous system, which is irrelevant to the severity of the tinnitus. *Tinnitus severity depends on the level of activation of the autonomic nervous system.*

> *Tinnitus severity depends on the level of activation of the autonomic nervous system.*

Autonomic Nervous System Activity

The sympathetic part of the autonomic nervous system is not an all-or-none system—it has different levels of activity. The highest (or most extreme) level is fight-or-flight. Low levels reflect a relaxed state. In between are moderate to high levels that are associated with stress.

Whether tinnitus becomes a problem for a person may depend on the level of activation of the sympathetic part of the autonomic nervous system at the time the

> A high level of activation of the sympathetic part of the autonomic nervous system may explain why tinnitus that emerges during a period of high stress can become such a problem.

person first experiences tinnitus. If the level of sympathetic activation is low, the person is more likely to naturally habituate to the tinnitus. If the level is high, then the tinnitus may further increase the activity—leading to the vicious circle encompassing awareness and reactions. A high level of activation of the sympathetic part of the autonomic nervous system may explain why tinnitus that emerges during a period of high stress can become such a problem.[64]

Conscious Loop

At the most basic level, activity in the limbic and autonomic nervous systems is controlled by two systems in the brain. One is the *conscious loop* that is dominated by conscious awareness. The other is the *subconscious loop* that involves subconscious processing of neural signals.

The conscious loop involves interconnections between the cortex, where conscious thought takes place, the limbic system, which mediates emotions, and the autonomic nervous system (Fig. 8-1). How we think about and respond to our tinnitus can be greatly affected by any fears associated with the tinnitus. Those fears can include concerns that the tinnitus reflects a brain tumor, impending deafness, or a mental disorder. Having fearful thoughts can ultimately affect the activity of the sympathetic part of the autonomic nervous system.

8-1. Conscious Loop. The conscious loop involves active connections between the auditory cortex, limbic system, and autonomic nervous system. (Figure adapted from Jastreboff and Hazell, 2004[4])

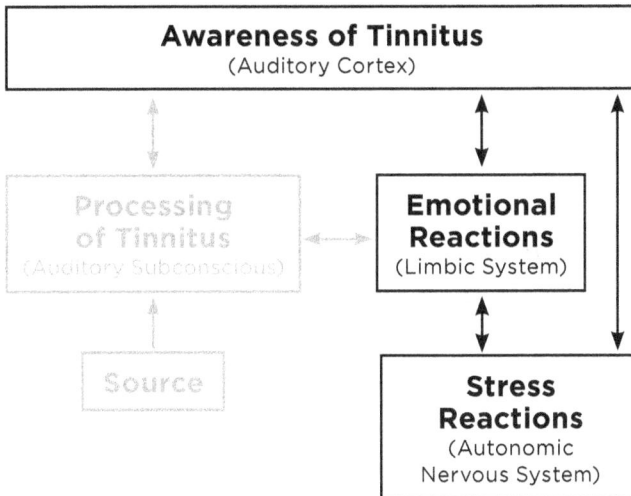

Subconscious Loop

The subconscious loop refers to interconnections between the limbic system, the autonomic nervous system, and subconscious areas of the auditory nervous system (Fig. 8-2). Conscious thinking is not a factor, but this loop can have the same, if not larger, effects on the limbic and autonomic nervous systems.

We discussed how, when tinnitus is bothersome, the tinnitus neural signal is linked to areas of the brain responsible for annoyance and stress. This link is the conditioned reflex. The subconscious loop is most generally caused by conditioned reflexes, which can result in chronic annoyance,

> For most people, a combination of conscious and subconscious loops is involved in causing the mental, emotional, and sleep problems associated with tinnitus.

anxiety, sleep disruption, and difficulty concentrating. They can even cause panic attacks that seem to occur out of nowhere. *All of these effects can be experienced without any conscious awareness of the tinnitus.*

For most people, a combination of conscious and subconscious loops is involved in causing the mental, emotional, and sleep problems associated with tinnitus. For anyone who is bothered by tinnitus, however, the subconscious loop is at least partially involved.

> **8-2. Subconscious loop.** The subconscious loop involves active connections between the limbic system, autonomic nervous system, and subconscious areas of the auditory nervous system. (Figure adapted from Jastreboff and Hazell, 2004[4])

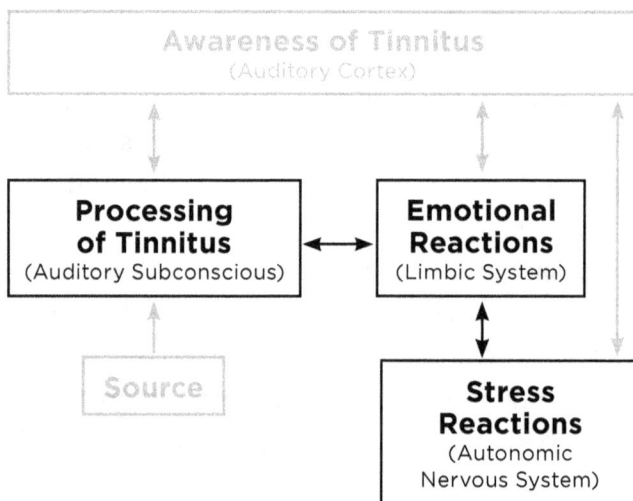

Reacting Constantly to Tinnitus

The subconscious loop may be more important than the conscious loop in causing the problems associated with tinnitus. The subconscious loop involves conditioned reflexes, which are learned (or conditioned) responses that occur automatically. The constant presence of tinnitus, whether the person is aware of it or not, can result in a constant *subconscious* reaction to the tinnitus. Tinnitus that is constant can be much more difficult to treat than tinnitus that occurs intermittently.

> The subconscious loop may be more important than the conscious loop in causing the problems associated with tinnitus.

Experiencing a New Sound

When a new sound is experienced, it activates the hair cells, auditory nerve, and auditory pathways up to the cortex. Because the sound is new, the auditory system gives it immediate attention, and the sound is evaluated in the cortex to determine its meaning. The new signal also evokes mild activity in the limbic and autonomic nervous systems.

Natural Habituation to a New Sound

If no action is required in response to a new sound, the signal will be classified by the brain as unimportant. Further exposure to the sound will result in a weakening of any reactive activity in the limbic and autonomic nervous systems. The sound will still be detected and processed by the auditory system, but it will not stimulate the limbic and autonomic nervous systems. *This is how habituation occurs to a meaningless signal—the signal is detected, but it does not reach conscious awareness.*

> This is how habituation occurs to a meaningless signal—the signal is detected, but it does not reach conscious awareness.

New Refrigerator

A new refrigerator serves as a good example of how you habituate naturally to some sounds. When a refrigerator is first installed, its sound is new to you and gets your attention. At first the sound may seem somewhat intrusive, which could result in slight annoyance and mild activation of your autonomic nervous system. The sound might even give the impression of malfunction, which could create anxiety and further activate your autonomic nervous system. Checking with the installer provides assurance that the refrigerator is functioning normally. That information addresses your concerns, and there is no reason to continue monitoring the sound—it's still there and it continues to activate your auditory nervous system, but you don't pay attention to it.

Classification of a New Sound: *Important*

In most circumstances, a new sound is immediately classified by the brain as *high priority* (a "10") relative to other sounds in the environment. There is awareness of the sound and some mild reaction. The sound is then evaluated to determine whether it (a) is important or unimportant, (b) indicates danger, and (c) indicates some action is needed.

Reclassification of a New Sound: *Unimportant*

To review, sounds such as a new refrigerator are quickly recognized as meaningless, resulting in the signal being classified by the brain as unimportant. Because of this classification, you are no longer aware of the sound most of the time, and the sound does not cause any annoyance even when you are aware of it.

How is this explained using the neurophysiological model? The *unimportant* classification of the sound caused the signal to be *filtered* at subconscious levels. Because of the filtering, the signal no longer maintains a connection with the limbic and autonomic nervous systems—meaning that any reactions to the sound have habituated. The filtered signal also does not normally activate auditory pathways up to the auditory cortex, meaning that habituation of the *perception* of the sound has taken place. Habituation of reactions and habituation of perception are the overall goals of TRT.

New Tinnitus

When tinnitus is first experienced, the brain evaluates it as for any new sound. Some people with new-onset tinnitus think the sound comes from somewhere in the environment. They may search for the source of the sound and even be convinced that there is a sound somewhere. Some people, referred to as *hummers*, think they hear low-frequency sounds coming from electrical transformers or gas pipes.[65] Most people, however, realize fairly quickly that their tinnitus perception stays the same as they move around the environment and between different environments. They know the sound originates within their head.

Habituation Occurs above the Tinnitus Generator

The *cure* for tinnitus would be to eliminate it at its source. The source of tinnitus is referred to as the *tinnitus generator—where the tinnitus neural signal is generated.* A cure is currently not available in spite of many years of intensive research. Finding a cure would mean discovering how the perception of tinnitus (the sound of the tinnitus) can be eliminated. That is something those of us with tinnitus all hope for. It is important to keep in mind, however, that tinnitus becomes bothersome not due to its perception but rather to reactions caused by the tinnitus.

> The source of tinnitus is referred to as the *tinnitus generator—where the tinnitus neural signal is generated.*

In the absence of an available cure, it is possible to habituate to the reactions caused by tinnitus. As we've discussed, these reactions are due to conditioned reflexes—tinnitus becomes bothersome when the tinnitus neural signal is linked to areas of the brain that are responsible for feelings of annoyance and stress. For treatment, this link needs to be broken—the conditioned reflex must be extinguished.

We pour water on a fire to put it out—to extinguish the fire. With TRT, we use special techniques to *extinguish the conditioned reflexes* that are associated with tinnitus—leading to habituation of reactions. This habituation process takes place *above the tinnitus generator* in the auditory nervous system. In other words, the tinnitus signal itself is unaffected (the tinnitus is still present) while the reactions are stopped (the tinnitus no longer impacts our sleep, concentration, or mood).

> This habituation process takes place *above the tinnitus generator* in the auditory nervous system.

Habituation taking place above the tinnitus generator helps to explain why measures of tinnitus loudness and pitch are not relevant to the distress caused by tinnitus. It also helps to explain how habituation can occur regardless of the cause or the diagnosis of tinnitus.

Main Goal of Treatment with TRT

Treatment with TRT has a *main goal* and a *secondary goal,* which are covered in these next two sections. Spoiler alert:

when you have reached the goals of treatment with TRT, you will stop reacting to your tinnitus (main goal) and will not be aware of it most of the time (secondary goal).

The main goal of treatment with TRT is habituation of your *reactions* to tinnitus. When this goal is reached, you would no longer have negative reactions to your tinnitus that are considered clinically significant. Importantly, the measures of tinnitus loudness and pitch made by the audiologist may not change when reaching the goal. Also, the percentage of time you are aware of your tinnitus may stay the same. In essence, the tinnitus should stop impacting your life even though you may still be aware of it.

> ...the tinnitus should stop impacting your life even though you may still be aware of it.

This main goal (habituation of the reactions to tinnitus) can be accomplished only by changing the functional connections (links) between the tinnitus signal in the auditory nervous system and the limbic and autonomic nervous systems (Fig. 8-3). Because of these connections, conditioned reflexes activate the sympathetic part of the autonomic nervous system.

> ...when at least partial habituation of reactions is achieved, your subjective perception of the loudness of your tinnitus should decrease...

It should be noted that when at least partial habituation of reactions is achieved, your subjective perception of the loudness of your tinnitus should decrease because of reduced input to the auditory nervous system from the limbic and autonomic nervous systems.

8-3. Habituation of Reactions to and Awareness of Tinnitus. Accomplishing the primary goal of treatment with TRT (habituation of reactions to tinnitus) leads automatically to accomplishing the secondary goal (habituation of awareness/perception of tinnitus). The graphic shows that full habituation involves tinnitus-related neural signals that are normally confined to the auditory system, below the level of awareness. (Figure adapted from Jastreboff and Hazell, 2004[4])

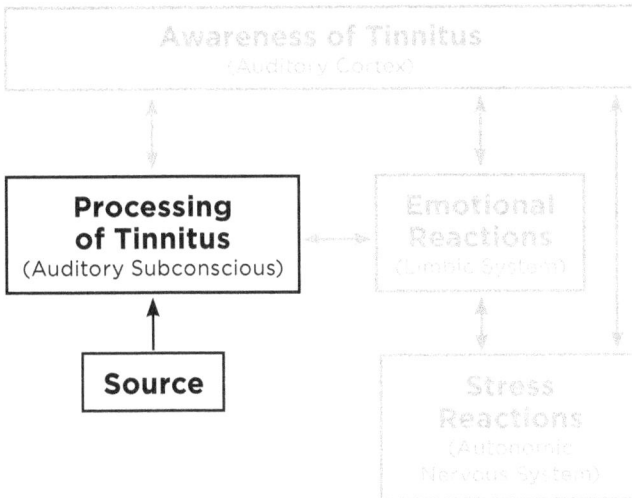

Awareness of Tinnitus
(Auditory Cortex)

Processing of Tinnitus
(Auditory Subconscious)

Emotional Reactions
(Limbic System)

Source

Stress Reactions
(Autonomic Nervous System)

Secondary Goal of Treatment with TRT

Habituation of the *perception* of tinnitus is the secondary goal of treatment with TRT. If you are unaware of the tinnitus all or most of the time (unless you purposely seek it), then the secondary goal has been met. Achieving this goal has nothing to do with changing the activity of the tinnitus signal in the auditory nervous system. What *does* change is that the tinnitus neural signal is normally blocked (filtered out) from reaching the auditory cortex, where it is consciously perceived (Fig. 8-3). This blocking of the neural signal occurs automatically once a sufficient level of habituation of reactions is achieved. In summary, accomplishing the primary goal of treatment with TRT leads automatically to accomplishing the secondary goal.

> ... accomplishing the primary goal of treatment with TRT leads automatically to accomplishing the secondary goal.

Habituation and Passive Extinction

We've discussed the learning process of habituation. We will now talk about *passive extinction*, which explains the habituation process in greater detail. We have also discussed the primary goal of TRT, which is *habituation of the reactions to tinnitus*. Another way of describing this primary goal is *passive extinction of conditioned reflexes*.

Passive extinction of conditioned reflexes was first described by the Russian scientist Ivan P. Pavlov.[66] We're going to dig deeper into these concepts about learning because they are essential to understanding how tinnitus habituation occurs.

As background, most people are aware of Pavlov's series of experiments with his "salivating dogs." His experiments demonstrated *classical conditioning*, meaning that a *meaningless stimulus* (the sound of a bell) can acquire the meaning of a separate, *meaningful stimulus* (food) by repeatedly pairing the sound of the bell with the delivery of food.[51] Without such pairing, the sound of the bell has no inherent meaning and elicits no response. The food *does* have an inherent meaning and elicits salivation (an *unconditioned response*—no learning needed). After pairing the bell with the food, the bell acquired the food's inherent meaning. The bell alone then elicited the same response (salivation) elicited by food (a *conditioned response*—learning required). These experiments demonstrated an *associative form of learning* where one stimulus acquires the same meaning as another stimulus because of the association between the two.

Can a conditioned response be *unlearned*? In the case of Pavlov's dogs, the bell caused a conditioned response because of its association with food. If the bell is then rung repeatedly but without food, the conditioned response will gradually be extinguished.[67] With extinction, the conditioned stimulus (the bell in this case) loses its ability to elicit the conditioned response (salivation) because of nonreinforcement (no food) of the conditioned stimulus (the bell). Put more simply, the bell lost its acquired meaning that food is present because food was no longer present when the bell was rung. The bell again became a meaningless stimulus, which is what it had been to begin with.

Passive Extinction of Conditioned Reflexes

Let's do a little review to make sure we are understanding the different terms being discussed. We just learned how a conditioned response can be extinguished if the reinforcement is no longer present. We refer to that process as *passive extinction*, which is essentially the same thing as habituation. We've also talked about conditioned responses, which we refer to as *conditioned reflexes*.

The neurophysiological model explains how the auditory nervous system is connected to the limbic and autonomic nervous systems. These connections have a subconscious loop and a conscious loop, which we discussed earlier (Figs. 8-1 and 8-2). The connections need to be modified, but there are no methods to modify them directly "because it is impossible to eliminate all reactions of the autonomic nervous system, which acts as a negative reinforcement. Therefore, a technique is used in which both the stimulus and the reinforcement are still present but decreased."[4] (p. 102) The technique is a specific method of passive extinction of conditioned reflexes.

More review: A meaningless stimulus (bell) acquires meaning when it becomes associated with some reinforcement (food). If the stimulus (bell) is presented repeatedly without the reinforcement (food), then passive extinction of the conditioned (or *learned*) reflexes (salivation) will take place. What is learned is that the stimulus (bell) is no longer associated with the reinforcement (food).

> It is not possible to eliminate all reactions to the tinnitus, which is why the classic method of passive extinction must be used in a modified fashion.

Now let's talk about how all this relates to tinnitus. The stimulus is the tinnitus signal, and the reinforcement, which is negative, is the reactions that take place in the autonomic nervous system. It is not possible to eliminate all reactions to the tinnitus, which is why the classic method of passive extinction must be used in a modified fashion. The modification used with TRT is to *reduce* (not eliminate) the negative reinforcement, while at the same time reducing the strength of the tinnitus signal by sound therapy, which we will discuss shortly.

Reclassification of Tinnitus

We are going use a specific method of passive extinction of conditioned reflexes to modify the connections between the auditory nervous system, limbic system, and autonomic nervous system (Fig. 7-2). For this method to work with tinnitus, we need to *reduce the reactions that occur in the autonomic nervous system in response to the tinnitus signal.* This is accomplished using four approaches.

First, it is necessary for the tinnitus signal to be reclassified at the cognitive (*thinking*) level as an

...we need to *reduce the reactions* that occur in the autonomic nervous system in response to the tinnitus signal. This is accomplished using four approaches.

First, it is necessary for the tinnitus signal to be reclassified at the cognitive (*thinking*) level as an unimportant (or neutral) stimulus.

unimportant (or neutral) stimulus. Reclassification of tinnitus to a neutral signal must occur in order for habituation to take place.

We discussed how tinnitus can be the side effect of normal compensation occurring within the auditory nervous system. One example of this is Dr. Jastreboff's theory of tinnitus generation based on discordant damage or dysfunction. *Discordant damage or dysfunction* refers to regions of outer hair cells being damaged or missing while inner hair cells are intact and fully functional. Tinnitus can occur as a side effect of compensation that takes place because of this discordant damage.

Another example of normal compensation was demonstrated by the Heller and Bergman experiment.[59] This experiment showed that tinnitus can emerge when people are placed in an extremely quiet environment, presumably causing enhancement of gain within the auditory nervous system.

What happens when tinnitus becomes reclassified as a neutral signal at the conscious level of the brain? This would indicate that the conscious loop affecting autonomic nervous system activity is either broken or the connections have been greatly reduced (Fig. 8-1). This also means that only the subconscious loop continues to activate the autonomic nervous system (Fig. 8-2).

Known Danger versus Unknown Danger

The second way to reduce autonomic reactions makes use of a psychological principle: *known danger causes much weaker reactions in the autonomic nervous system than unknown danger.* As an example of how this principle works, a dental patient will be less anxious about an upcoming procedure if the steps of the procedure are clearly explained—compared to receiving no explanation. With TRT, we follow this principle by explaining possible mechanisms responsible for tinnitus perception and reasons why tinnitus causes

> The second way to reduce autonomic reactions makes use of a psychological principle: *known danger causes much weaker reactions in the autonomic nervous system than unknown danger.*

negative emotional reactions. The framework for explaining these concepts is the neurophysiological model. Gaining an understanding of these concepts can reduce the activity in the autonomic nervous system that is linked to the tinnitus neural signal.

Thinking Positively about Tinnitus

The third way to reduce autonomic reactions is to establish new associations for tinnitus with positive thoughts and ideas. Rather than thinking about tinnitus in negative terms, we can think about it in positive terms, such as "Tinnitus is the music of the brain."

> The third way to reduce autonomic reactions is to establish new associations for tinnitus with positive thoughts and ideas.

Positive thoughts and feelings of hope will result

in reduced activity in the autonomic nervous system. Treatment with TRT is all about achieving success, and we have good reason to believe that success is likely. Many clinical reports have demonstrated successful results with TRT.[4] As described in appendix A, research has shown that TRT is effective for most patients, and it is even more effective for patients with the greatest tinnitus severity.[68-75]

Stress Management

The fourth way to reduce activity in the autonomic nervous system is to reduce your overall stress level. Most people with bothersome tinnitus lead very stressful lives, both at work and at home. These stresses contribute to the overall level of activity in the autonomic nervous system. It is therefore helpful to use any reasonable method of stress management.

> The fourth way to reduce activity in the autonomic nervous system is to reduce your overall stress level.

There are more formal and less formal methods of stress management. More formal methods include relaxation training, biofeedback, massage, and hypnosis. Less formally, being organized, managing time efficiently, and participating in various recreational activities can

> Stress management by itself, however, is generally insufficient to achieve permanent habituation of tinnitus.

reduce stress. Many different stress management methods can contribute to weakening feedback loops that are responsible for maintaining a high level of annoyance in response to the tinnitus signal. Stress management by itself, however, is generally insufficient to achieve permanent habituation of tinnitus.

Review the Four Methods to Reduce Activity in the Autonomic Nervous System

1. The tinnitus signal must be reclassified at the conscious level of the brain as an unimportant (or neutral) stimulus.
2. Make use of the psychological principle: *known danger causes much weaker reactions in the autonomic nervous system than unknown danger.*
3. Establish new associations for tinnitus with positive thoughts and ideas.
4. Reduce your overall stress level.

What about Distraction Techniques?

A method that is commonly used to get relief from tinnitus is distraction, using various means to shift attention away from tinnitus and onto other things. These strategies may be helpful in the short term, but they also may be counterproductive with respect to achieving long-term habituation of tinnitus.

Directing attention away from tinnitus is effective only if a person is actively thinking about the tinnitus. It does

> Directing attention away from tinnitus is effective only if a person is actively thinking about the tinnitus.

not affect connections between the auditory nervous system and the limbic system. If those connections are causing activity in the autonomic nervous system, being distracted will result in no change in the connections, and habituation of the reactions to tinnitus will not occur. Distraction techniques may even have the opposite effect of attracting attention to the tinnitus.

Sound Therapy

We've discussed various techniques for achieving passive extinction of conditioned reflexes to tinnitus. None of these techniques involves the therapeutic use of sound, which we'll now cover. TRT uses a specific method of *sound therapy* to facilitate extinction of conditioned reflexes.

Counseling and sound therapy are the two essential components of treatment with TRT. The purpose of sound

> The purpose of sound therapy is to *decrease the strength of the tinnitus signal*.

therapy is to *decrease the strength of the tinnitus signal*. It does not require the use of any particular device. It is, however, important that any device used for sound therapy produces high-quality sound and that the sound is comfortable and non-annoying.

Reducing Contrast = Reducing Strength

Our *sense organs* enable awareness of our immediate environment. We sense touch and pain by *tactile receptors* that cover the body. We sense different smells by *olfactory receptors* in the nose. We see what's around us because of *photoreceptors* in our eyes. And we hear sounds around us because of the hair cells (*mechanoreceptors*) in our inner ears. When we are active, we are literally flooded with sensory information, which we will refer to as *stimuli*.

Each *stimulus* is detected by a sense organ, and the body is "wired" to evaluate the importance of the stimulus and whether some action is required. One of the features of each stimulus is its strength. A stimulus has *absolute* strength (that can be measured) and *relative* strength (compared to the strength of competing stimuli). Our focus here is on relative strength.

The relative strength of a stimulus depends on the *contrast* between the stimulus and the background, which is referred to as the *figure-ground relationship*. In this book, for example, printing the words in black against a white background creates maximum contrast so that the words are easy to read. Another example is a candle flame. The flame seems bright in a dark room (maximum contrast) but not as bright with the lights on (reduced contrast) (Fig. 7-5).

The tinnitus neural signal is a stimulus, and like all stimuli, one of its features is its strength. Like the candle in the dark room compared to having the lights on, the relative strength of the tinnitus neural signal depends on the background neural activity (Figs. 7-5 and 7-6). If the background neural activity is low (high contrast), then the tinnitus neural signal seems stronger. If the background neural activity is increased (less contrast), the strength of the tinnitus neural signal is perceived as weaker.

Sound therapy for TRT is based on the principle that the strength of the tinnitus neural signal depends on the background neural activity in the auditory system. Sound in the environment increases that background neural activity, which *reduces the contrast* between the tinnitus-related neuronal activity and the background activity. Here's the relevant question: According to the neurophysiological model, what does reducing the contrast do?

Reducing the contrast between the tinnitus-related neuronal activity and the background activity has two results with respect to the conscious and subconscious loops that we discussed earlier (Figs. 8-1 and 8-2). First, reducing the contrast *reduces the strength* of the tinnitus signal that connects to the cortical and limbic areas of the brain. Second, reducing the contrast means that detection of the tinnitus signal by subconscious neural networks becomes more difficult. The tinnitus signal is therefore *less detectable* by these networks. Reducing the detectability of the tinnitus signal facilitates the process of habituation, both of the reactions to and the perception of tinnitus.

> Reducing the contrast between the tinnitus-related neuronal activity and the background activity has two results with respect to the conscious and subconscious loops...

Suppression of Tinnitus Is Counterproductive to Habituation

We are returning to the topic of suppression of tinnitus. Recall that when we talked about the mixing point, I explained that the term *masking* is typically used to refer to the use of sound to change or cover up the sound of tinnitus. With TRT we refer to *suppression* rather than masking to more correctly describe what takes place in the brain when external sound changes or covers up the sound of tinnitus.[5,51] We discussed how a sound can cause complete suppression, partial suppression, or no suppression.

No suppression means the sound you hear has no effect on the sound of your tinnitus. A sound that results in no suppression is below the mixing point, which is where you want it for sound therapy with TRT. Sound that causes either partial suppression (changing the sound of the tinnitus) or complete suppression (eliminating the perception of the tinnitus) is what is typically used to achieve temporary relief

> A sound that results in no suppression is below the mixing point, which is where you want it for sound therapy with TRT.

from tinnitus (either of these effects is how the masking method works[76]). Partial or complete suppression of tinnitus, however, is counterproductive to facilitating tinnitus habituation. Why is it counterproductive?

Partial or complete suppression of tinnitus means the sound of the tinnitus has changed or is gone altogether. *Habituation of tinnitus requires the sound of the tinnitus to be unchanged.* The objective is to habituate to the tinnitus that is *normally experienced* and not to some modified version of the tinnitus. More technically, extinguishing conditioned reflexes requires that the stimulus (the tinnitus) be present with its usual characteristics to learn that that particular stimulus (the tinnitus) is not reinforced. According to this basic principle, therefore, the extinction procedure for retraining the brain to habituate to tinnitus requires that the tinnitus signal be unchanged.

> Habituation of tinnitus requires the sound of the tinnitus to be unchanged.

Prescription Medications and Tinnitus

Many people take prescription medications for their tinnitus. Most of these types of drugs target the central nervous system for management of anxiety, which means they act to reduce activity in the limbic and autonomic nervous systems. No drug, however, has been shown to be consistently effective for tinnitus, and there is always the concern of negative side effects.[12,14,77]

The recommendation with TRT is that no prescription drug should be taken specifically for tinnitus unless an emergency situation requires it or if a person has coexisting mental health issues requiring pharmacological management. If a person is taking medications, any treatment for tinnitus must be carefully coordinated with the prescribing physician. It's important to keep in mind that positive results from TRT can also result in a significant reduction in anxiety and depression without the use of mood-altering medications.

Drugs Can Impair Learning

The use of medications during treatment with TRT can slow the process of habituation if they impair central nervous system plasticity. This is especially a concern for benzodiazepines, which are known to affect the central nervous system.[78] Benzodiazepines can theoretically interfere with the ability to modify conditioned reflexes and to participate in the mental and learning activities that are necessary with TRT.

If you are taking any prescription medications, you should *not* stop taking them when treated with TRT. Any decision about medications should be made by your prescribing physician. If you do speak with your physician, you might ask about medications that do not impair memory, such as drugs that act on glutamate receptors, calcium channels, and sodium channels.

Habituation Takes Time

Let's review some points so that you have realistic expectations about when to expect habituation to take place. The primary goal of treatment is habituation of tinnitus reactions. Achieving this goal requires retraining the limbic and autonomic responses that are linked to the tinnitus signal. We are using a specific method of passive extinction of conditioned reflexes to modify these connections. Extinction of conditioned reflexes ideally would remove the negative reinforcement. As we discussed, with tinnitus the negative reinforcement cannot be removed completely during this process.

Achieving even partial habituation normally requires months because retraining occurs slowly and gradually. When will you know that partial habituation has occurred? It may be so gradual that you won't realize the process has started. During follow-up visits your progress may become apparent when you answer the questions on the Follow-up Interview. Follow-up visits also help us to be most efficient in reviewing the important concepts and making any changes to treatment that might be necessary.

When partial habituation of reactions is achieved, you might notice that the loudness of your tinnitus seems to have decreased. I explained that this can occur because of reduced input to the auditory nervous system from the limbic and autonomic nervous systems.

Most people experience partial habituation within the first six months of treatment. Some people experience improvement within one or two months. Regardless of your rate of progress, follow-up visits should be repeated every few months for at least 12 months to prevent relapse. If more than 12 months are needed, treatment continues until no further help is desired. During treatment you may notice periods of rapid progress and periods of seemingly no progress. Regardless, the TRT protocol should be followed closely to optimize your progress.

> Most people experience partial habituation within the first six months of treatment.

Summary

We've gotten through all of the counseling material. It's a lot of information, and it will be important to continue to review it so that the concepts taught can facilitate the changes that need to be made to lead to habituation.

There are seven main summary points:

1. The perception of tinnitus is the result of normal compensation of the auditory system to some dysfunction or damage (typically in the cochlea). This damage can even be as subtle as the ordinary loss of hair cells over time through natural attrition.

2. Perceiving tinnitus is not a problem in itself. It becomes a problem only if it *causes negative emotional reactions.*

3. Negative reactions caused by tinnitus are due mainly to conditioned reflexes.

4. Treatment with TRT is designed to retrain conditioned reflexes. Retraining results in habituation of the reactions caused by tinnitus and habituation of the perception of tinnitus.

5. For habituation to occur, the brain must reclassify the tinnitus neural signal as a neutral, or meaningless, signal.

6. The proper use of sound therapy assists in the habituation process by *decreasing the strength* of the tinnitus signal.

7. The primary goal of TRT is habituation of the reactions caused by tinnitus. When the primary goal is achieved, habituation of the perception of tinnitus follows automatically, which is the secondary goal of TRT.

CHAPTER 9

Follow-up Visits

The treatment described thus far is for category 1 and 2 patients. Category 0 patients require less counseling while still covering the main points. Category 3 and 4 patients require specific modifications to the ongoing treatment protocol (described in appendixes D and E, respectively).

Ongoing treatment is essential to perform TRT properly. All patients should be followed as necessary to ensure that they are fully compliant with every element of the treatment protocol. They also need to maintain an awareness of the principles of TRT counseling, which requires reviewing the counseling on a repeated basis over the course of treatment.

I will now explain why ongoing treatment is important, and I'll describe the follow-up visit schedule and what's done during the visits. After that, I will ask the questions from the TRT Follow-up Interview to see how well you're doing with treatment. We will review the key counseling points to make sure you still have a good understanding of the concepts. Finally, I'll provide suggestions to address any concerns that may arise about not making progress and to determine the end point of treatment.

Why Ongoing Treatment Is Important

TRT counseling involves repeated educational sessions. Many new and technical concepts are introduced. People have different abilities to retain new information, but in general, anyone receiving treatment with TRT needs the counseling repeated so that the concepts can become established in their minds. It is a well-known principle that learning is maximized through repetition.

In case you're interested, studies have shown that people remember only about 50% of the information received through educational counseling.[79,80] Much of the information may be remembered incorrectly,[79] and as much as 80% of the information can be forgotten immediately.[81] For these reasons, many TRT clinicians provide take-home handouts to review the counseling information between visits.

My research group completed a study that supports the need for ongoing treatment (the study is described in appendix A).[69,82] In that study, participants made return visits at 3, 6, 12, and 18 months. The counseling was reviewed at each visit, and measures were repeated to determine whether

> Treatment progress actually may be minimal during the first six months of treatment, with the *greatest effects occurring after six months.*

progress had been made. The average responses of the TRT participants to these test measures showed a consistent progression of improvement at each subsequent visit. Treatment progress actually may be minimal during the first six months of treatment, with the *greatest effects occurring after six months*. These results suggest that for TRT counseling to be most effective, it should be repeated at intervals over a period of at least a year (except for category 0 patients, who require only minimal counseling).

Follow-up Visits

A general rule of thumb is to attend follow-up visits at four weeks, three months, six months, and then every six months until treatment is no longer needed.[44,46] Exceptions to this schedule may be necessary for anyone who needs a greater amount of attention or for those who are unable to make so many repeat visits. If travel poses a problem, counseling should at least be performed remotely (via telephone or online video meetings) at the recommended intervals.

You completed your four-week and three-month follow-up visits. At every visit we started by checking your hearing aids for normal functioning, and we reviewed your use and adjustment of the sound generators to ensure that you have been using them properly. At the four-week visit we finished going through all of the counseling, which took us an hour and a half. At the three-month visit we spent two hours asking the questions from the Follow-up Interview and reviewing all of the counseling. We also did a basic hearing test.

Today's visit is your six-month appointment, which should take up to two hours. We will do everything we did at your three-month appointment. We will not do tinnitus loudness and pitch matching because you have not reported any changes in what your tinnitus sounds like. We also will not repeat testing your loudness discomfort levels because you do not have a sound tolerance problem. At each visit, counseling time is progressively reduced as you become increasingly familiar with the information.

TRT Follow-up Interview

The questions from the TRT Follow-up Interview are asked at all follow-up visits.[11,51] The Follow-up Interview contains a subset of questions from the Initial Interview. Some questions are essentially the same between the initial and follow-up versions but are modified for the follow-up version to determine how well you are doing with your treatment.

Instructions for Completing the Follow-up Interview

When I ask these questions from the Follow-up Interview, please think about your tinnitus and its effects over the previous month when you answer each question. You should not respond in relation to any particular day or circumstance; think about how the tinnitus has affected you *generally* during the past 30 days. With each question we want to determine whether there has been an improvement in your condition.

Tinnitus

We will first ask questions specific to your tinnitus. Please think only about your tinnitus when you answer these questions.

> **Question 1. Do you have "bad days" when your tinnitus is more bothersome than usual, or does it seem equally bothersome from day to day? *If yes*, do you have these bad days more often, less often, or just as often as you did before you started treatment? *If yes*, are your bad days the same, not as bad, or worse than before you started treatment?**

The question about the number of bad days is asked in the Initial Interview (question 7), and additional questions were added to the Follow-up Interview to determine whether the number of bad days has changed relative to baseline. With positive results of treatment, people will report fewer bad days than before. When answering these questions, it is important to know if you are taking any mood-altering medications, which could definitely affect whether you consider a day to be good or bad.

With positive results of treatment, people will report fewer bad days than before.

Your personal response to this question from the Initial Interview was that your days when tinnitus was more bothersome than usual seemed to be associated with stressful relationships, especially when dealing with interpersonal conflict. You have worked on that, and you have felt less stressed overall. You now experience bad days less frequently, which is generally what we would expect from anyone who is working on reducing their stress.

> **Question 2. Do sounds ever cause a change in the loudness of your tinnitus?** *If louder,* **what kinds of sounds cause this change? When any of these sounds cause your tinnitus to change, how long does the change last? When you hear a sound that causes your tinnitus to change, does the effect sometimes last until the next morning after you've slept?** *If yes,* **what kinds of sounds cause this to happen?**

These questions were asked from the Initial Interview to determine whether you might be a TRT category 4 patient. If so, that would mean that certain sounds cause your tinnitus to become louder and the increased loudness continues until at least the next morning. This is an uncommon condition, and we determined that you would not be a category 4 patient. According to your responses today, it is still not a concern, so we continue to treat you as a category 2 patient.

> **Question 3. Do you use ear protection (earplugs or earmuffs)?** *If yes,* **why do you use protection? Do you use it specifically because of the tinnitus?** *If so,* **what percent of the time do you use earplugs or earmuffs** *for your tinnitus***? Do you use earplugs or earmuffs** *for your tinnitus* **when it's fairly quiet?**

These questions are to determine whether you might be overprotecting your ears with earplugs or earmuffs. The concern is that overprotecting your ears could make you more sensitive to sound and potentially even increase the perceived loudness of your tinnitus.

> ...overprotecting your ears could make you more sensitive to sound and potentially even increase the perceived loudness of your tinnitus.

During the Initial Interview you said that you never used hearing protection. That certainly meant that you were *not* overprotecting your ears. It did, however, raise the concern that you might not be using hearing protection when needed to protect your ears from loud sound that could be damaging. We discussed that concern, and you've reported today that you carry earplugs with you and use them whenever sound seems loud enough to cause damage. A good rule of thumb is, if sound in your environment is so loud that

> ...if sound in your environment is so loud that you must raise your voice to be heard by a person standing next to you, then it is too loud for you.

you must raise your voice to be heard by a person standing next to you, then it is too loud for you.

Question 4. Are you currently receiving any other treatment specifically for your tinnitus? *If yes*, what?

The point of this question is to make sure you are not receiving any treatment for your tinnitus that might conflict with what we're doing with TRT. You have been advised to enrich your sound environment 24/7 for sound therapy, so any use of sound that is comfortable and non-annoying is acceptable. Otherwise, you are not receiving any other treatment for your tinnitus, so you are on track to continue with TRT.

Question 5. What is the *biggest reason* your tinnitus is a problem (not including trouble hearing or trouble understanding speech)?

It is particularly important to compare your response to this question with your original response from the Initial Interview. The "biggest reason" that tinnitus is a problem can change from visit to visit, and the focus of treatment may need to be modified accordingly to address what you feel is your current primary concern.

When we originally asked this question, you said the biggest reason your tinnitus was a problem was that it keeps you awake at night. You were advised to add sound to your sleep environment, and you purchased a bedside sound generator. The bedside device has lots of different sounds, and you've been experimenting with the options. Apparently, you like some of the water sounds, and you've been using them to provide comfortable background sound during your sleep time. Sleep continues to be the biggest reason your tinnitus is a problem, so it is appropriate to continue experimenting with different sounds.

Question 6. I'm going to read through a list of activities, and I want you to tell me how often your tinnitus keeps you from doing these activities or how often it negatively affects these activities in any way. Please don't include trouble hearing or trouble understanding speech when you answer these questions.

This is a follow-up question to determine the impact of tinnitus on your various life activities. I have your responses to the Initial Interview, so I can directly compare your responses between then and now. It's best if you don't know your previous responses to help ensure that your responses today are independent and unbiased.

	Never	Rarely	Some-times	Often	Always	N/A
Concentration?	☐	☐	☐	☐	☐	☐
Sleep?	☐	☐	☐	☐	☐	☐
Quiet resting activities (reading, relaxing, etc.)?	☐	☐	☐	☐	☐	☐
Work? (select N/A if retired)	☐	☐	☐	☐	☐	☐
Day-to-day responsibilities outside of work?	☐	☐	☐	☐	☐	☐
Going to restaurants?	☐	☐	☐	☐	☐	☐
Participating in or observing sports events?	☐	☐	☐	☐	☐	☐

	Never	Rarely	Some-times	Often	Always	N/A
Social activities?	☐	☐	☐	☐	☐	☐
Anything else?	☐	☐	☐	☐	☐	☐

I can tell you that your sleep, which was your biggest problem, has improved somewhat. The other activities that were affected before treatment were concentration, work, and social activities. According to your responses today, you are showing improvement in all of these areas. Sleep deprivation affects every aspect of life, so because you're getting better sleep it's not surprising that you're doing better overall.

Question 7. What percent of your *total awake time*, over the last month, were you *noticing or thinking about* your tinnitus? Please give an average percentage over the last month. Has this percentage changed since the beginning of treatment? *If yes*, how much do you think it has changed?

Question 8. What percent of your *total awake time*, over the last month, were you *annoyed, distressed, or irritated* by your tinnitus? Please give an average percentage over the last month. Has this percentage changed since the beginning of treatment? *If yes*, how much do you think it has changed?

Questions 7 and 8 directly address the main goals of treatment, which are habituation of perception and habituation of reactions, respectively, to tinnitus. You are being asked to estimate the percentage of your awake hours, over the previous month, that you were aware of your tinnitus (consciously thinking about it) and annoyed by your tinnitus (reacting to it emotionally). These percentages will decrease over time if treatment is successful in achieving habituation.

Your percentages were fairly high at the beginning of treatment. We are looking for the percentages to go down gradually as treatment progresses. For both questions, you were asked, "Has this percentage changed since the beginning of treatment? *If yes*, how much do you think it has changed?" Sometimes responses to these additional questions contradict the actual differences in percentages between the Initial and Follow-up Interviews. Usually, when this happens, people are unaware of how much of a reduction has taken place over the course of treatment. When such a discrepancy occurs, this would be pointed out to emphasize the amount of progress that has been made. In your case, the percentages have dropped, and you are consistent in estimating how much they have dropped.

> **Question 9. How *strong*, or *loud*, was your tinnitus, on average, over the last month? "0" would be "no tinnitus"; "10" would be "as loud as you can imagine."**

When we completed the Initial Interview, we discussed how tinnitus loudness cannot be directly measured. The loudness of sounds in the environment can be measured with a decibel meter, but the loudness of tinnitus

...the loudness of tinnitus is a wholly subjective experience.

153

is a wholly subjective experience. People with tinnitus typically describe its loudness with respect to how much they are bothered by it.[36,47] If they are bothered more, the tinnitus can seem louder. If they are bothered less, it can seem softer. These kinds of reported changes in tinnitus loudness cannot be verified by any measurement procedure.

All that being said, if you think your tinnitus has become softer, that's an indication of improvement. Today you are reporting that your tinnitus loudness is a "5," which is definitely less than what you reported prior to treatment.

Question 10. How much has tinnitus *annoyed you*, on average, over the last month—not including annoyance from trouble hearing or trouble understanding speech? "0" would be "not annoying at all"; "10" would be "as annoying as you can imagine."

This is a key question to determine how you are progressing toward the main goal of TRT, which is habituation of emotional reactions due to tinnitus.[4,5] *Annoyed* is the word used in the question, but it could just as well be *bothered, distressed,* or *irritated.*

Without mentioning the actual number you chose when we did the Initial Interview, I can say that it was very high. Your number today of "5" shows a significant improvement. Consistent with the goal of TRT, we are working toward getting that number down even further.

Question 11. How much did tinnitus *impact your life*, on average, over the last month—not including impact from trouble hearing or trouble understanding speech? "0" would be "not at all"; "10" would be "as much as you can imagine."

The previous question addressed your emotional reactions to tinnitus. This question expands on the previous one to ask how your life in general has been affected (impacted) by tinnitus. As I mentioned during the Initial Interview, this is really a quality-of-life question. How much has tinnitus affected your quality of life over the past month?

Your response today to this question is what I would have expected based on your other responses to the Follow-up Interview. You chose a "5," and that is a significant improvement compared to how you answered the question from the Initial Interview.

Question 12. Do you have any other comments about your tinnitus?

During the Initial Interview you expressed concern that your tinnitus cannot be cured and that all we are doing is managing it. Management did not feel like an acceptable solution to you, and you were skeptical that treatment would make any difference. You were, however, willing to keep an open mind and give it a try. Your response today is that you are encouraged that treatment really does make a difference. Treatment is not yet complete, but you know you are making progress and believe you will continue to make progress.

We've completed the Tinnitus portion of the TRT Follow-up Interview. The next section asks about your ability to tolerate sound. You did not report this to be a problem before, but we need to ask again to make sure it is not currently a problem.

> ## Question 13. Are sounds bothersome or unpleasant to you when they seem normal to other people around you? *If yes*, what kinds of sounds are bothersome or unpleasant?

You responded that you now have a better understanding of the intent of this question. It's asking if you are uncomfortable with sound that does not cause discomfort for other people. This was not a problem for you then, and it is not a problem now. For anyone who reports a sound tolerance problem, there are more questions to better understand the problem. Those questions are described in appendix D. We can now move on to the question about your hearing.

> ## Question 23. Do you think you have a hearing problem?

> It is important at every visit to determine whether you feel that you have a hearing problem.

It is important at every visit to determine whether you feel that you have a hearing problem. The key concern is your *perception* of a hearing problem, regardless of the results of any auditory testing.[83] This perception can change between appointments. Category 1 patients do not report a hearing problem during the initial assessment, but after using sound generators they may report their hearing has since become difficult in some circumstances.[82] For this reason, it may be preferable to fit hearing aids with built-in sound generators (combination instruments) rather than using sound generators alone. Combination instruments, however, are much more expensive than sound generators alone. Many TRT clinicians therefore do not start out with combination instruments unless they feel that amplification will likely be required at some point.

Your hearing problem was made evident during your evaluation visit. Because of that, you are being treated as a category 2 patient, meaning you have a significant problem with both your tinnitus and your hearing. You have been wearing hearing aids, and you now report that your hearing is still a problem—but only a slight one.

> **Question 24. How much of a problem is _tinnitus_ (if you are not including problems from trouble hearing or trouble understanding speech)?** "0" would be "no problem at all"; "10" would be "as much as you can imagine."

You rated your tinnitus problem as a "5," which is again consistent with your other responses and indicates that you are making improvement.

Question 25. How much of a problem is *trouble tolerating sound*? "0" would be "no problem at all"; "10" would be "as much as you can imagine."

Your previous response indicated a slight sound tolerance problem because of your concern that sound could make your tinnitus worse. Your response today was zero because you are aware that while some sounds can be so loud as to cause damage to your ears, everyday sounds do not carry that risk. You now make that distinction and carry earplugs with you as insurance against such loud sounds. Otherwise, you have no worries about tolerating the usual sounds in your environment.

Question 26. How much of a problem is *hearing*? "0" would be "no problem at all"; "10" would be "as much as you can imagine."

We just confirmed that you still have a hearing problem, but it is mostly remedied by wearing hearing aids. You have been wearing hearing aids, and you now report that your problem hearing is a "1" on the zero-to-ten scale.

While hearing aids are helpful, they are not like glasses, which are able to completely restore normal vision for most people. Hearing difficulties are usually only partially corrected by hearing aids. It is therefore not expected that you would report a zero, which would mean your hearing is "no problem at all."

> Hearing difficulties are usually only partially corrected by hearing aids.

Question 27. Next I would like you to tell me if you are doing the same, better, or worse with each of the issues we have talked about.

	Same	Better	Worse	N/A
Tinnitus	☐	☐	☐	☐
Trouble tolerating sound	☐	☐	☐	☐
Hearing	☐	☐	☐	☐

If you combine those issues, would you say your problem in general is the same, better, or worse than before you started treatment?

Problem in general	☐	☐	☐	☐

In response to this question, I'm glad to know that you feel you are doing better with your tinnitus and your hearing difficulties. You are making good progress with your tinnitus, which was your primary complaint. You are having less of a problem with your hearing thanks to the hearing aids. You realized that sound tolerance really wasn't a problem to start with, and you stated that your sound tolerance problem was "better" simply because you now understand what a sound tolerance problem refers to. Given the improvement in each of these areas, it is not surprising that you feel that your "problem in general" is better.

Question 28. How would you feel if you had to give back your instruments?

☐ They don't seem to be helping but I'd be unhappy/upset about giving them back because I'd like to keep trying.

☐ They don't seem to help and returning them wouldn't bother me.

☐ They seem to be helping and I'd be unhappy/upset if I had to return them.

☐ They seem to be helping but returning them wouldn't bother me.

This question is to determine your true feelings about your combination instruments. Some patients are adamant (or defensive) in stating that they would not want to give up their instruments. The question often generates a discussion about the effectiveness of the devices, which can be helpful to both patient and clinician. You chose the response "They seem to be helping and I'd be unhappy/upset if I had to return them."

Your combination instruments are working well for you. The hearing aid portion is helping you to hear better, which mostly addresses your hearing problem. You have been using the sound generators according to the proper protocol, and they seem to be helping to facilitate habituation to your tinnitus.

Question 29. Are you glad you started this program?

☐ No   ☐ Yes   ☐ Not sure

This final question in the TRT Follow-up Interview simply asks if you are glad that you started treatment. Your "yes" response provides a further indicator of the overall effectiveness of treatment.

Tinnitus Questionnaire

We also had you complete the Tinnitus Functional Index during this appointment. Your score of 76 before treatment indicated a "severe" problem with tinnitus. Your score today of 42 might be considered a "moderate" problem with tinnitus. Based on the eight subscale (domain) scores, the areas where you were having the most trouble before treatment were emotional reactions, sleep, and ability to concentrate. You have shown improvement in each of those areas. You are definitely making progress.

Counseling Review

Please keep in mind that the purpose of the counseling is for you to reclassify your tinnitus so that it will become a benign, meaningless sound. This reclassification is necessary to start the process of habituation and also for your sound therapy to be effective.

We have spent considerable time talking through all of the counseling. We discussed each concept in detail, and you were able to understand the information. Today we will review each of the main topics using a list of questions that I developed. This is a long list, and it will not be easy to answer many of the questions even though all of the counseling has been completed—and repeated. Even experienced TRT practitioners might have difficulty answering many of the questions. This list can also be used as a handout to take home to review the topics. The topics generally follow the order of the counseling that is described in chapters 7 and 8. Page numbers where the answers can be found are listed after each question.

- What is the *mixing point* and why is it important for sound therapy? (page 71)
- What is *discordant damage or dysfunction* of hair cells and how might that underlie tinnitus? (page 91)
- What is *auditory gain* and how does it change to adjust to the level of ambient sound? (page 93)
- What was the Heller and Bergman experiment,[59] and how did it show that almost everyone has tinnitus under certain circumstances? (page 94)
- How does *the cocktail party effect* relate to being aware of tinnitus even in the midst of background sound? (page 96)
- How does the *candle in a dark room* analogy explain how the strength of a signal varies depending on the surrounding signals? (page 97)
- Why is it important to *avoid silence* and maintain some background sound? (page 99)
- What do *automated responses* have to do with managing sensory overload? (page 100)
- How are *important* and *unimportant* signals managed differently by the brain? (page 101)
- What does it mean that *signals are prioritized according to their relative importance*? (page 102)
- What is *brain plasticity* and why is it important for treating tinnitus? (page 103)
- Can conditioned reflexes be *retrained*? Can they be *extinguished*? (page 103)

- What are the roles of the *auditory nervous system,* the *limbic system,* and the *autonomic nervous system?* (page 104–105)
- What part of the brain is responsible for the *fight-or-flight* response? (page 106)
- How is *chronic stress* different from the fight-or-flight response? (page 107)
- How are *tinnitus* and *chronic stress* related? (page 108)
- When we hear a sound that *does not cause an emotional reaction,* what part of the brain is activated? (page 111)
- If sound *does* cause an emotional reaction, what major parts of the brain are activated? (page 111)
- What is different about the *sympathetic* and *parasympathetic* parts of the autonomic nervous system? (page 107)
- What does the *vicious circle* refer to? (page 44)
- Why do people often experience an enhanced perception of their tinnitus during sleep time? (page 113)
- Can prescription medications help to break the vicious circle? (page 113)
- Does louder tinnitus cause greater tinnitus distress? (page 114)
- The *severity of tinnitus* is affected by which part(s) of the brain? (page 114)
- The *conscious loop* involves interconnections between what areas of the brain? (page 116)
- The *subconscious loop* involves interconnections between what areas of the brain? (page 117)

- Are both the *conscious* and *subconscious loops* active in causing problems due to tinnitus? (page 117)
- When a person hears a *new sound,* does it evoke activity in the limbic and autonomic nervous systems? (page 119)
- What learning process describes how a new sound can be detected but not reach conscious perception? (page 119)
- What happens to our awareness of the sound of a new refrigerator? (page 120)
- When a sound no longer maintains a connection with the limbic and autonomic nervous systems, what has been habituated? (page 121)
- Is it possible to habituate to both the *reactions to* and the *perception of* tinnitus? Can one lead to the other? (page 123)
- Habituation of what aspect of tinnitus is the *main goal* of TRT? (page 123)
- Habituation of what aspect of tinnitus is the *secondary goal* of TRT? (page 125)
- Do *habituation* and *passive extinction* refer to the same learning process? (page 126)
- Are emotional reactions to tinnitus a conditioned reflex? (page 103)
- If a stimulus is presented repeatedly without reinforcement, what takes place? How does this relate to tinnitus? (page 126–127)
- Why is *reclassification of tinnitus to a neutral signal* important? (page 129)
- How does the principle that *known danger causes weaker reactions in the autonomic nervous system than*

unknown danger pertain to being counseled about the neurophysiological model of tinnitus? (page 130)

- Do *positive thoughts and feelings of hope* affect activity in the autonomic nervous system? (page 131)
- Is *good stress management* usually sufficient to achieve permanent habituation of tinnitus? (page 132)
- Do *methods of distraction* contribute to long-term habituation of tinnitus? (page 133)
- Which component of TRT has the purpose of *decreasing the strength of the tinnitus signal?* (page 134)
- Why does the strength of the tinnitus neural signal depend on the background neural activity? (page 135)
- Does *partial or complete suppression* (masking) of tinnitus facilitate tinnitus habituation? (page 137)
- Has *any drug* been shown to be consistently effective for tinnitus? (page 138)
- Is it OK to take *benzodiazepines* during treatment with TRT? (page 139)
- How many months of treatment with TRT are necessary for most people to experience some habituation? (page 139)

If You Feel Like You're Not Making Progress

If people feel they are making minimal or no progress during treatment, it's usually because they are unaware that they have been making gradual progress over time.[51] Progress is often so gradual that it is imperceptible on a

> Progress is often so gradual that it is imperceptible on a day-to-day basis.

day-to-day basis. Responses to questions from the Follow-up Interview will then reveal that progress actually has been made. Some patients, however, will in fact not make progress, which will be confirmed by their questionnaire and interview responses. If little or no progress has been made after about one year of treatment, the clinician must make a full assessment of what might be hindering progress.

Some possible reasons for treatment failure include:[4]

1. The person was assigned to the wrong treatment category, resulting in inappropriate treatment.
2. Symptoms were temporarily worsened shortly after treatment started, and the person was not properly counseled as to why this might have happened.
3. The person did not fully comprehend the counseling information, and thus reclassification of tinnitus to a neutral stimulus did not occur.
4. The neurophysiological model was not taught properly.
5. Follow-up appointments were not made or were inadequate.
6. Significant psychological problems were untreated.
7. Medications taken for psychiatric illness worsened the tinnitus or impaired the brain's plasticity, which is necessary for habituation.

8. The person is involved in litigation or is somehow receiving secondary benefit from the tinnitus (for example, workers' compensation benefits).
9. The person has a need to attract attention (*flag-wavers* describes patients who use their tinnitus or decreased sound tolerance as a pretext to attract attention).

Each of these possibilities needs to be considered for the person who is not showing progress. Obviously, these factors need to be checked and addressed properly at the beginning of treatment.

Importantly, there is evidence that better health outcomes are associated with adherence to the treatment protocol.[84] Treatment compliance is also a responsibility of the clinician; that is, the clinician must ensure that the patient returns for counseling sessions according to the recommended treatment schedule. Patients also need to be questioned carefully to make sure that they are using their ear-level devices according to the protocol.

I personally observed some participants from a controlled study who reported that they were not making progress through about one year of treatment with TRT, but they continued to comply with the protocol, and significant improvement was seen during the last period of treatment.[82] Some people thus need to be encouraged to continue the treatment protocol in spite of their apparent lack of progress.

> In general, progress tends not to be linear, but more typically has hills and valleys.

In general, progress tends not to be linear, but more typically has hills and valleys.

The majority of people mainly want their tinnitus to be completely eliminated. The lack of a cure should be discussed prior to the start of treatment; otherwise, the person being treated may never be satisfied.

A decrease in the perception of tinnitus loudness is generally observed in people who successfully achieve even partial habituation of tinnitus. The neurophysiological model predicts this phenomenon as a side effect of decreased feedback from the limbic and autonomic nervous systems on the auditory nervous system.[85] (Also, loudness matches of tinnitus may remain the same after treatment.) Should the perception of tinnitus loudness fail to be reduced, treatment can still be considered a success if and when significant habituation of reactions and perception is achieved.

Determining the End Point of Treatment

Treatment is complete when everyone agrees that treatment is no longer necessary. Making this decision is helped by how you respond to the questions in the TRT Follow-up Interview. Your responses should indicate that tinnitus is no longer a significant concern. You should not, however, stop using your sound generators at the time you first realize that you no longer require treatment. In this case, you would be advised to continue using your sound generators for at least two to three months to ensure that the retraining that has taken place is permanent.[4]

Treatment would, of course, be ended if you were no longer compliant with the follow-up schedule of appointments or with the protocol for using your devices. When treatment is complete, you will be advised to use your sound generators as needed in the future should your tinnitus ever increase or worsen. In the case of combination instruments, a similar procedure is used for the sound generator portion of the instruments. Practically all people with hearing aids will continue to use their hearing aids, but they are instructed that there is no need to provide additional sound enrichment as required during treatment.

Achieving habituation of reactions and perception will empower you to withstand and overcome potential future tinnitus fluctuations. Any "spiking" of your tinnitus or your reactions to it may cause a renewed sense of concern and necessitate further evaluation and counseling. If this occurs, then habituation of reactions and perception can usually be achieved at a faster pace.

PART 4

Wrap-up

CHAPTER 10

Summary, Suggestions, and Resources

Summary

We might think of tinnitus as a *real sound that is not associated with a sound wave*. The perception of tinnitus is the reality. It's there in our heads, but it does not exist anywhere else. For most of us with tinnitus, the sound is constant no matter where we are or what we're doing. It's our "traveling companion" of sorts, and not necessarily a welcome one.

Many people with tinnitus do not pay attention to it most of the time—they habituate to it just like they habituate to sounds in their environment that are not relevant to what matters to them. Unfortunately, some people with tinnitus can't help but pay attention to it much of the time. Continually paying attention to tinnitus can be part of the vicious circle of awareness → reactions → awareness. The problem is not the tinnitus sound itself but the reactions to it. Once the vicious circle has taken root, it is difficult to undo and can greatly impact a person's quality of life. The process of learning to react less to the tinnitus (habituation of reactions) automatically results in paying less attention to the tinnitus (habituation of perception). Facilitating this learning process is the purpose of TRT.

Although the underlying neural mechanisms of tinnitus are not fully understood, we have many insights from what is known about how sounds are processed in the brain. By applying this knowledge, different aspects of how tinnitus is processed in the brain can be reasonably theorized. The neurophysiological model describes tinnitus as neural activity in the auditory nervous system that can involve other parts of the central nervous system (cortex, limbic system, and autonomic nervous system) when tinnitus is bothersome. These other parts of the brain are involved in the vicious circle that progressively enhances the tinnitus neural signal. Retraining the limbic and autonomic responses is how TRT is designed to break this vicious circle and block the tinnitus signal from reaching cortical areas of awareness.

Achieving the goals of TRT largely depends on how well the clinician delivers the counseling and directs the sound therapy. As already mentioned, it can be difficult to find a competent tinnitus practitioner, whether for TRT or any other method of treatment. Most of these methods involve some form of counseling combined with sound therapy.[86] In spite of any claims you might have heard, there is no proof that any one method is superior to the others. In defense of TRT, our controlled clinical trial showed that treatment with TRT, when done properly by a trained and experienced professional, can be effective for the majority of patients treated.[69,82] The research evidence for TRT is reviewed in appendix A.

Although it is essential to conduct TRT according to the specified protocol, in reality many clinicians greatly shorten the counseling, do not properly implement the sound therapy, and do not provide the needed follow-up care. TRT practitioners should be fluent in describing the neurophysiological model and able to answer the review questions about TRT listed in chapter 9. They should practice TRT with minimal variation to ensure that every patient receives the same standard of treatment.

With study and experience in performing TRT according to the protocol, clinicians can become proficient TRT practitioners. The effectiveness of TRT also depends on clinicians being compassionate, unhurried, and concerned with the whole person rather than trying to "fix" an isolated problem. Ultimately, the goal is to empower patients so that they can gain control over how they react to tinnitus and reach a point of relief and a lifestyle unhindered by tinnitus.

Suggestions to Optimize Success with TRT

These suggestions are adapted from previous publications. [3,87]

1. Learn as much as you can about TRT on your own (additional resources listed below).
2. Work with a competent TRT provider.
3. Understand tinnitus and its benign nature.

4. Fully understand the neurophysiological model of tinnitus and how it is used to reclassify tinnitus to the category of a neutral stimulus.

5. Continue to review the TRT review questions listed in chapter 9.

6. Avoid silence and maintain an enriched environment of low-level, comfortable sound—even when sleeping.

7. If wearing sound generators (or hearing aids with a sound generator):

   a. Use two devices—one in each ear.

   b. At the start of the day, adjust the first sound generator to just below the mixing point. This is done by turning up the volume of the sound very gradually to the level at which the sound of the tinnitus starts to change—this is the mixing point. Then turn the volume down *just slightly*. The second sound generator is adjusted to the same loudness as the first. It is important that the sound of the tinnitus remains unchanged while the sound therapy makes it less detectable (promoting habituation). It is also important that the sound generators are set so that within a few minutes the sound they produce is neither annoying nor distracting.

   c. Use your wearable devices during all waking hours without readjusting them after they are set at the start of the day. The point is to "set and forget" the devices to minimize paying attention to your tinnitus.

8. Attend follow-up visits as often and as long as necessary.
9. Be patient. Stick with the program.

TRT Resources

Any website, video, or articles from Drs. Pawel and Margaret Jastreboff; also any articles or information from Jonathan Hazell, Susan Gold, and Jacqueline Sheldrake.

Websites for Stephen M. Nagler, MD, FACS and Atlanta Tinnitus Consultants, LLC (www.atlantatinnitus.com) (www.tinn.com); access to articles, interviews, Q&A, and information consistent with the principles of TRT; Dr. Nagler is also available to provide telephone and Skype consultation.

Michael J. A. Robb, MD (www.RobbMD.com); Robb Oto-Neurology Clinic, Phoenix, Arizona; 20 years specializing in diseases and disorders of the ear and the brain; co-author of two TRT books published in 2007.[10,51]

Gail B. Brenner, AuD (tinnitus-philadelphia.com); Dr. Brenner has been a TRT practitioner since the mid-1990s.

The original book describing TRT: *Tinnitus Retraining Therapy: Implementing the Neurophysiological Model.*[4]

Word-for-word (scripted) TRT counseling in the present book is based directly on the contents of the original TRT book.[4] The scripted counseling has been adapted from a previous book that I authored.[51] My previous book was written for professionals, while the current book is written for the general population of people who experience tinnitus. A companion flip-chart counseling book is available that corresponds topic-by-topic with the counseling script.[10]

Concluding Thoughts

It's been a pleasure for me to be your *virtual clinician* and to walk you through the different stages of TRT. We have stuck to the protocol through your six-month visit, and I've pointed out the progress you have made. You still have more to do, but I have every reason to believe that you will be mostly habituated to your tinnitus within the next six months or so. We've talked about how habituation takes time, and you're in the middle of that learning process taking place in your brain. Please keep up with the sound therapy, periodically review the counseling points, and stay hopeful for continued progress. I'll see you at your next visit!

PART 5

Appendixes

APPENDIX A

What Is the Evidence for TRT?

To determine whether a method of treatment works for *any* medical condition, we rely mostly on *randomized controlled trials*. A randomized controlled trial is a research study that gives a treatment to one group of people and compares the results to a *control* group (that receives a different treatment or no treatment). For TRT, there are many clinical and research studies but relatively few randomized controlled trials. In my previous book,[3] appendix G ("How Do We Know If a Treatment Works?") describes how we rely mostly on randomized controlled trials, systematic reviews, and meta-analyses to determine the strength of evidence for any method of treatment.

In the present appendix, I review randomized controlled trials that have been conducted to evaluate TRT. These kinds of trials provide the highest confidence that the results reflect a true effect (relative to studies that are nonrandomized and uncontrolled).[88] It needs to be pointed out, however, that even if a study is randomized and controlled, the study may have flaws that could affect (or *bias*) the results.

Placebo Control

In a randomized controlled trial, *placebo control* is ideal so that study participants don't know if they are receiving the treatment or not. Some studies, such as drug-treatment studies, can use a placebo-control group, but TRT and other *habituation-oriented* methods of tinnitus treatment (such as cognitive behavioral therapy, Progressive Tinnitus Management, and Tinnitus Activities Treatment) generally cannot. And keep in mind that these approaches treat *effects* of tinnitus, such as sleep problems, concentration difficulties, and emotional reactions. They can decrease your awareness of tinnitus, but they cannot completely eliminate your tinnitus.[3]

Recruitment and Enrollment

A randomized controlled trial must enroll people who would be appropriate candidates to receive the treatment being tested. Finding such people is the *recruitment* process. Candidates are recruited to enroll in the trial *if they are qualified*. Qualified candidates for evaluating a method of tinnitus treatment would be people who have bothersome tinnitus and could benefit if the treatment were to make their tinnitus less bothersome (there are, of course, numerous other requirements). A person meeting the study requirements (and who is willing to participate) is enrolled and randomized to either receive the treatment being studied or belong to a control group.

Systematic Reviews

A number of randomized controlled trials have been completed to evaluate different methods of tinnitus treatment. Many of these trials have undergone a process called *systematic review*. A systematic review looks at all of the randomized controlled trials that are relevant and determines which ones meet certain quality standards. Those meeting the standards are evaluated according to a number of criteria and then rated for their *strength of evidence*. Based on this information, the overall benefit of the particular treatment is assessed and reported in the scientific literature.

A systematic review was published in 2014 that included "nine high-quality studies" for both TRT and cognitive behavioral therapy (CBT).[68] Eight of the trials assessed CBT relative to a no-treatment control group, and one evaluated TRT compared to tinnitus masking. The authors of this systematic review concluded, "both therapies resulted in significant improvements in quality of life scores. . . . Both CBT and TRT are effective for tinnitus, with neither therapy being demonstrably superior."[(p. 1028)]

Many more systematic reviews have been done to evaluate methods of treatment for tinnitus. We can't review them all here, but we can highlight a few that are representative of the overall conclusions: (1) CBT has the strongest body of evidence.[89] (2) There is no evidence that sound therapy *on its own* provides significant benefit.[90] (3) Regarding hearing aids, there is "currently no evidence to support or refute their use as a more routine intervention for tinnitus."[91] (p. 2)

Clinical Practice Guidelines

Systematic reviews are also used to develop *clinical practice guidelines,* which provide recommendations for what to do and what not to do to address a health condition. Prior to 2017, four clinical practice guidelines for tinnitus had been published in Europe and one in the United States. All five of these clinical practice guidelines were reviewed, summarized, and reported in 2017.[12] The following is a very brief summary of the tinnitus treatment recommendations across all five guidelines: (1) Educate patients about tinnitus and options for management. (2) Use hearing aids only if warranted for hearing loss. (3) CBT should be offered to patients with bothersome tinnitus. (4) Medications and dietary supplements should *not* be used. In addition to these recommendations, there was a lack of agreement regarding the use of sound-based therapy.

The 2017 review of clinical practice guidelines for tinnitus[12] did not recommend any treatment except CBT. In 2023, another review of tinnitus practice guidelines was published.[92] In the newer review, six sets of guidelines were identified. These were from the US (2014), Switzerland (2019), Europe (2019), Great Britain (2020), Germany (2021), and Japan (2019). All six sets of guidelines reviewed in 2023 support treatment with CBT. None of them support phar-macological treatment (including prescription medications and dietary supplements). Regarding TRT, the review con-cludes that various studies have shown improvement but the quality of evidence was low, with a high risk of bias. They note that it has been debated whether sound therapy contributes to the effects of TRT.

Based on the conclusions of these two reviews of tinnitus practice guidelines,[12,92] why would anyone want to receive TRT? I will do my best to answer that question, which raises some controversial issues. Ultimately, it should be *your informed decision* whether you believe TRT can be effective for treating bothersome tinnitus.

Randomized Controlled Trials for TRT

Henry et al. (2006)

I attended formal TRT training in 1997. I received additional training years later to stay up-to-date with any changes to TRT. After my initial training, I wrote a grant proposal to evaluate TRT compared to tinnitus masking. That study was funded and 123 research participants were enrolled.[69,82] Each participant attended five counseling sessions over 18 months. They all wore ear-level devices, which included dif-ferent makes and models of hearing aids, tinnitus maskers (sound generators), and masker/hearing aid combination instruments. I personally performed the TRT counseling one-on-one with 64 of the participants. The other 59 partic-ipants were counseled by an audiologist who was skilled in the tinnitus masking method.[93]

Both groups showed substantial and approximately equal improvement for the first 6 months. At 12 and 18 months, the TRT participants showed further improvement, while those in the masking group maintained their same level of improvement (they seemed to plateau). It was concluded, "TRT may have its greatest effects after 6 months of treatment, thus treatment with TRT should be conducted in a longitudinal manner to achieve optimal benefit."[69] (p. 69)

This TRT trial was evaluated in a systematic review.[94] The review concluded, "TRT was beneficial in the management of tinnitus but this support for the intervention must be tempered by the limited and low quality of evidence."(p. 8) The only criticism of the study was the method by which participants were assigned to treatment groups: "The first qualifying patient was placed into a treatment group by random selection. Each subsequent qualifying patient was placed by alternating between groups."[82] (p. 107) The reviewers considered this method of alternating assignment to constitute "allocation bias," meaning the possibility that results could be affected because it was always known what treatment group the next participant would be assigned to. We responded to that concern in 2022: "In this trial, the audiologist who assessed candidates for eligibility was not aware of the randomization order and was not one of the investigators who delivered treatment; these details were not stated in the article."[88] (p. 2334)

Another systematic review came to a similar conclusion about our TRT trial as well as five other trials that were eligible for review, stating, "The quality of the studies was generally low."[90] (p. 11) In our defense we argued, "The judgments rendered by these two Cochrane reviews effectively discredited the results of a controlled clinical trial that showed significant benefit with both TRT and tinnitus masking."[88] (p. 2334) We further pointed out that, because of the Cochrane review conclusions, TRT is not recommended in clinical practice guidelines "and consequently may not be offered to patients who could benefit from their use."[88] (p. 2334)

In our article in which we defended our TRT trial, we came to the overall conclusion, "These reviews become critiques of research methodology and the effectiveness of the intervention is marginalized or 'beside the point.' Unfortunately, the conclusions of a systematic review can make it appear that an intervention for tinnitus is not effective, even if the opposite is true. All told, the tinnitus-related systematic reviews have concluded that all tinnitus management strategies, other than CBT, have low-quality evidence. . . . The results of this process have had a deleterious effect on guidelines that have been published for tinnitus clinical management."[88] (p. 2337)

Henry et al. (2007)

This randomized controlled trial evaluated the TRT counseling delivered to groups of participants.[70] Participants did not receive the assessment nor the sound therapy components of TRT. For the trial, 269 military Veterans with bothersome tinnitus were randomized into one of three study arms: TRT counseling, traditional support group, and no treatment. I personally conducted the counseling for 94 participants, who each attended four weekly 90-minute group sessions. Participants completed questionnaires through 12 months.

Overall, the TRT counseling group showed significantly more benefit than either the traditional support group or the no-treatment group. In spite of these favorable findings, it was determined that participants would have done better if they had undergone a formal TRT assessment, received hearing aids if needed for hearing loss, and used wearable sound generators if needed for severe tinnitus. To my knowledge, this randomized controlled trial of TRT group treatment has not been evaluated in a systematic review.

Westin et al. (2011)

Sixty-four participants with normal hearing were randomized into one of three groups: TRT, acceptance and commitment therapy (ACT), and wait-list control.[71] The TRT participants attended a 2.5-hour session and a 30-minute follow-up session, and they used ear-level sound generators for 18 months. The ACT participants attended 10 weekly 1-hour sessions. Overall, ACT was significantly more beneficial than TRT or than being on a wait list.

Tyler et al. (2012)

This trial compared three versions of TRT.[72] All three groups received the same picture-based counseling, which the authors developed to have a "heavy emphasis on neurophysiology." Participants completed follow-up questionnaires at 12 months.

Group 1 attended three clinic visits (45 to 60 minutes each) of counseling only. The other two groups also used ear-level sound generators, and they attended four clinic visits. For group 2, the sound generators were adjusted to totally mask (make inaudible) the tinnitus. For group 3, the sound generators were adjusted to the mixing point (defined for this study as the minimum level of noise that started to "mix" or "blend" with the tinnitus). Group 3 was the closest to what was recommended by the developers of TRT.[4]

A total of 48 participants completed the study. Participants showing improvement (defined as at least a 20% reduction in their tinnitus questionnaire score) at 12 months included four of the 20 participants in group 1 (counseling), six of the 13 in group 2 (total masking), and nine of the 24 in group 3 (mixing point). Overall effectiveness across all groups was "moderate to large." There were no significant differences between the three groups.

Henry et al. (2016)

This was a multisite randomized controlled trial conducted at four Veterans Affairs medical center sites.[73] Participants were 148 Veterans who were randomized into one of four groups at each site: TRT, tinnitus masking, tinnitus educational counseling (and hearing aids if needed), or a wait-list control group. The three treatment groups received comparable time and attention from audiologists, and the treatment schedule for participants in all three treatment groups followed the TRT protocol (visits at baseline and 3, 6, 12, and 18 months).

The three treatment groups all showed significant improvement, and no one treatment was more effective than the others. Without treatment, the wait-list control group did not show significant change. It was noted that "TRT did not exhibit the clear advantage in outcomes relative to tinnitus masking at 12 and 18 months as was previously found."[73] (p. e357) This lack of superiority might be explainable because "The previous study used tinnitus experts with many years of experience. The follow-up (present) study used audiologists who were mostly inexperienced with tinnitus; training was very limited; and half of the sites had high turnover of audiologists."(p. e358)

Bauer et al. (2017)

For this randomized controlled trial, all 38 participants attended three 1-hour counseling sessions and were followed for 18 months.[74] Nineteen participants received TRT and 19 received "standard of care treatment."

The TRT counseling covered Jastreboff's neurophysiological model, mechanisms of hearing, and "how hearing loss and emotional reactions lead to bothersome tinnitus."[73] (p. 169) The TRT sound therapy used combination instruments—hearing aids with a built-in noise generator—with the noise set to a volume that was "audible and comfortable . . . but less loud than their tinnitus."(p. 169) The group receiving standard of care treatment used hearing aids along with counseling on "mechanisms of hearing, hearing health, coping, and listening strategies."(p. 169)

Both groups had a significant reduction in their tinnitus severity within 6 months, which was sustained for 18 months. Some measures showed a greater improvement for the TRT group. The authors concluded, "Both TRT and standard of care, as defined in the present study, provided lasting therapeutic benefit to individuals with chronic bothersome tinnitus. TRT, however, appeared to be somewhat more efficacious."[(p. 175)]

Scherer & Formby (2019)

A randomized, placebo-controlled trial was conducted at six United States military hospitals with 151 participants randomized to one of three study groups.[75] The three groups were full TRT (TRT counseling and ear-level sound generators for sound therapy), partial TRT (TRT counseling and placebo sound generators), and standard of care ("a patient-centered counseling protocol that aligned with current military care and recommended practice guidelines"[(p. E3)]). The counseling and fitting of devices followed the basic principles of TRT.[4] The placebo sound generators presented noise for 40 minutes, which was then reduced gradually to no output.[75]

Overall, all three groups showed similar results—there were no significant differences between any of them. The authors noted a number of limitations that could have affected the findings. First, there was a large number of missed visits and withdrawals in the full TRT and partial TRT groups, possibly due to participant frustration caused by sound generator problems early in the study. Second, there was a "lack of study clinician expertise in providing TRT at study outset. None of the study clinicians was initially proficient with, or routinely provided, TRT."[(p. E7)] In spite of these

limitations, each of the treatments resulted in "clinically significant improvement in most treated individuals."[p. E9]

Summary and Conclusions

There are different schools of thought on how to evaluate
methods of treatment for tinnitus. The most accepted
viewpoint scientifically is to consider conclusions from systematic reviews and clinical practice guidelines as having
the greatest validity. In this appendix, systematic reviews
and clinical practice guidelines were summarized, with
the overall conclusion that CBT has the strongest evidence
based on randomized controlled trials. Paradoxically, very
few CBT clinicians know anything about tinnitus.

We reviewed randomized controlled trials that have been
completed for TRT. If you've read through the summaries
of each trial, then you know that they were all conducted
differently and very different results were obtained. It
is impossible to compare the different studies—they are
"apples and oranges." Because of the inconsistency in how
these studies were conducted, systematic reviews cannot
accomplish a fair evaluation of the effectiveness of TRT.

From my perspective, TRT has substantial evidence
based on my professional experience with TRT. I was
funded as the principal investigator for three randomized controlled trials that evaluated TRT (total of over $1.5
million in grants from Veterans Affairs Rehabilitation,
Research & Development Service). I am the first author
for seven articles about TRT published in peer-reviewed
journals.[9,11,19,69,70,73,82] I am the lead author for two books on

TRT,[10,51] seven more articles about TRT in trade journals, and over a dozen presentations about TRT at national and international conferences, which included professional training seminars.

As I've stated elsewhere in this book, if you are considering evaluation and treatment with TRT, it is essential that your clinician (usually an audiologist) is fully trained and competent in delivering TRT. Ask the clinician, When and where were you trained? Did you attend the Jastreboff training? How long have you been conducting TRT? Do you follow the TRT protocols that are described in the TRT books?[4,10,51] How many patients have you treated with TRT? What evidence do you have that your patients have benefited from treatment with TRT?

APPENDIX B

Medical History

The AAO-HNSF published their "Clinical Practice Guideline: Tinnitus" in 2014.[14] The purpose of the guideline was "to provide evidence-based recommendations for clinicians managing patients with tinnitus. . . . It will discuss the evaluation of patients with tinnitus, including selection and timing of diagnostic testing and specialty referral to identify potential underlying treatable pathology."(p. S1)

One of their recommendations was that "clinicians should perform a targeted history and physical examination at the initial evaluation of a patient with presumed primary tinnitus to identify conditions that if promptly identified and managed may relieve tinnitus."(p. S1) In this appendix, we will review their suggestions for performing a "targeted history" (medical history). It is beyond the scope of this book, however, to review the details of a physical examination, which is a medical assessment performed by an otolaryngologist or other ear-specialist physician. The full AAO-HNSF guideline is available as a free-access article to view online (https://journals.sagepub.com/doi/full/10.1177/0194599814545325).

Medical History

The otolaryngologist's (or other ear-specialist physician's) role is to "identify potentially treatable causes of tinnitus as well as to identify serious conditions that may cause tinnitus or accompany tinnitus. An appropriate clinical evaluation should occur early to direct the need for and the type of additional testing and treatment."[14] (pp. S9-S10) The physician looks for potential causes of *secondary tinnitus*, which the AAO-HNSF defines as "tinnitus that is associated with a specific underlying cause (other than sensorineural hearing loss) or an identifiable organic condition."(p. S3)

A simpler way of thinking about secondary tinnitus is that it is "sound vibrations in the head," as opposed to primary tinnitus, which is "nerve activity in the brain."[3] The AAO-HNSF stated, "Although these causes of secondary tinnitus should be evaluated and managed, exclusion of these disorders is necessary to identify the patients with primary tinnitus that are the focus of this clinical practice guideline. In addition, the patient encounter should identify any severe coexisting mental illness, such as depression or dementia, as these patients may need expedited referral and management."[14] (p. S10)

It should be mentioned that some clinicians have a problem considering any kind of tinnitus to be related to sound vibrations. To their way of thinking, all tinnitus is subjective tinnitus. *Objective tinnitus* (and anything related to actual vibrations) would be *somatosounds* (that is, not tinnitus at all).

We will review briefly below the key concerns that a clinician must be aware of when conducting a medical history with patients complaining of tinnitus. These concerns are "symptoms and conditions that dictate the need for referral to otolaryngology, audiology, and related specialties."[14] (p. S10)

Sudden Onset of Hearing Loss

Sudden onset of hearing loss (with or without tinnitus) is considered a medical emergency that should be evaluated within 24 hours by both an audiologist and an otolaryngologist.[14,43] Otolaryngology treatment may need to start immediately. Specific guidelines regarding sudden hearing loss were published in 2019 by the AAO-HNSF.[95]

Unilateral Tinnitus

Unilateral tinnitus is tinnitus in one ear (or one side of the head) only. This raises the concern of a lesion (any kind of abnormality or tissue pathology) on the tinnitus side, such as a tumor (either benign or malignant/cancerous).[26,27] Unilateral tinnitus indicates the need for a medical assessment by an otolaryngologist and a comprehensive hearing evaluation by an audiologist.[14] Additional testing, such as imaging, might also be needed. It is worth noting that such tumors are relatively rare, even among individuals with unilateral tinnitus.

Unilateral or Asymmetric Hearing Loss

Unilateral or asymmetric (more on one side than the other) hearing loss raises the same concern as for unilateral tinnitus; that is, the possibility of a lesion, especially a tumor, on the affected side.[14]

Pulsatile Tinnitus

Pulsatile tinnitus (tinnitus that pulses with the heartbeat) raises the concern of problems with the cardiovascular system (heart and blood vessels).[96,97] A cardiovascular examination should be conducted, along with examination of the head and neck to look for vascular tumors or other related problems. Comprehensive audiology should be performed, and additional tests, such as imaging, might be needed.

Recent-Onset Tinnitus

Recent-onset tinnitus is tinnitus that has been present for less than six months.[14] It is distinguished from sudden-onset tinnitus, which often occurs with sudden-onset hearing loss (as described above). Recent-onset tinnitus is considered to be more *labile* than persistent tinnitus (present for at least six months), meaning the tinnitus "may diminish or disappear, and/or tinnitus reactions may be reduced."[14] (p. S10) Further evaluation and the potential for treatment are based on the severity of the condition, as well as the presence of any other symptoms.

Noise Exposure

Noise exposure during occupational and recreational activities is commonly associated with the onset and worsening (exacerbation) of both hearing loss and tinnitus.[98,99] Exposure to loud noise has the potential to damage the inner ear (cochlea).[100] It is important to be aware of this cause-and-effect relationship so that you know to take measures to protect your ears from any future loud noise.[14]

Medications and Potential Ototoxic Exposures

Ototoxic refers to anything that has the potential to damage the inner ear or central auditory system. This term is used mostly in relation to drugs and medications with this potential. Ototoxicity is mostly a concern with certain medications that would be administered in a hospital (usually the chemotherapy drug cisplatin and the aminoglycoside antibiotics).[101,102] These drugs are well known to cause hearing loss and tinnitus.[103] Over-the-counter medications can also trigger tinnitus, which is usually temporary. Salicylates (aspirin) can cause temporary tinnitus but generally only at higher doses.[100] Importantly, "interactions between medications have unknown effects and can exacerbate tinnitus symptoms.[14] [(p. 10)] Counseling regarding medication use is important and should include a list of known ototoxic medications.

Dizziness or Vertigo

Dizziness and vertigo have been defined by other authors[104] [(p. 2)] as follows: "Dizziness is the sensation of disturbed or impaired spatial orientation without a false or distorted sense of motion.[105] Vertigo, on the other hand, is a specific type of dizziness defined as the sensation of self-motion when no self-motion is occurring or the sensation of distorted self-motion during an otherwise normal head movement.[105]"

Experiencing dizziness or vertigo can indicate a disorder of the auditory nervous system, including the inner ear.[14] These disorders include Ménière's disease (experienced as intermittent vertigo, hearing loss, and tinnitus[106]), superior canal dehiscence (an abnormal opening in one of the three fluid-filled bony loops in the inner ear called semicircular canals, which sense rotations of the head[107]), and vestibular schwannoma (tumor on the eighth/auditory nerve, which connects the inner ear to the brain stem[108]). To determine whether any of these or other related disorders are present in someone experiencing dizziness or vertigo, a vestibular (balance) assessment is needed, which may include imaging, by an audiologist and ear-specialist physician (otologist, otolaryngologist, etc.).[14]

Symptoms of Depression and/or Anxiety

Depression and anxiety are common among tinnitus clinic patients according to numerous studies.[109-112] These symptoms may be preexisting (prior to the tinnitus), or they may be a consequence of having tinnitus. Either way, it is important to identify the potential for these conditions to be present in patients.[14] Screening instruments are available for this purpose. To screen for anxiety and mood, the Generalized Anxiety Disorder Scale-7 can be used.[113-115] The Patient Health Questionnaire-9 (PHQ-9) can be used to screen for depression.[116,117] Patients who screen positive for these conditions need to be referred to mental health professionals for assessment and possible treatment.[14]

Although not mentioned in the AAO-HNSF guideline,[14] it is also important to screen for insomnia. In fact, insomnia has been credibly reported as the most common effect of bothersome tinnitus.[31,118] The Insomnia Severity Index (ISI) is a valid assessment tool to assist in the evaluation of insomnia complaints.[119] The ISI has also been shown to be sensitive to treatment response in clinical patients.[120] Addressing insomnia is a critical concern for many patients who receive clinical services for tinnitus. Treatment for bothersome tinnitus may be sufficient to mitigate the insomnia. Some patients, however, require referral to a practitioner who specializes in managing sleep problems.

Apparent Cognitive Impairments

Cognitive impairments have been associated with tinnitus in numerous studies.[121-124] This association could be due primarily to two factors.[124] First, concentration difficulties are one of the main complaints of tinnitus patients, and these difficulties could be reflected in any test of cognitive performance. Second, the prevalence of both tinnitus and cognitive decline increase with age; therefore, the two conditions are loosely correlated. There is no evidence of a *causal* relationship between cognitive skills and tinnitus-related distress.

Elderly tinnitus patients are at risk for cognitive decline from dementia, which could affect assessment results and compliance with any treatment requirements.[14] It therefore may be important to screen for cognitive impairment in these patients. Many screening instruments are available for this purpose. One of the most popular is the Mini-Mental State Examination, which is appropriate for screening elderly patients.[125]

APPENDIX C

Audiological Evaluation

Audiologists are hearing healthcare professionals who specialize in evaluating and managing hearing problems. They usually have an audiology doctorate (AuD) degree, which is the current requirement, while others have a master's degree in audiology—the previous requirement.[126]

Because up to 90% of people with tinnitus also have hearing loss,[127] anyone with tinnitus should have an audiological evaluation.[128] As part of the evaluation, audiologists can determine whether hearing aids would be helpful. If so, audiologists are qualified to dispense hearing aids.

Audiologists and Tinnitus Management

Because there are no educational standards regarding tinnitus, audiologists receive different types and amounts of training in tinnitus management.[129] Fortunately, some AuD programs provide substantial training.[130] Otherwise, audiologists have the opportunity to receive tinnitus training from conference presentations, workshops, and online courses.

One option for audiologists is to complete the Certificate Holder–Tinnitus Management (CH-TM) training program developed by the American Board of Audiology (ABA) (https://eaudiology.audiology.org/tinnitus). When audiologists have "CH-TM" after their name, that means they have completed this training and earned the CH-TM certificate. The certificate indicates that certain knowledge has been gained but does not guarantee competence in tinnitus management. If requesting tinnitus services from an audiologist, it is important to ask about any training received and the amount of experience providing tinnitus clinical services.

Audiological Evaluation for TRT

Before any testing is done, the audiologist will use an otoscope to look in your ears and make sure your eardrums look good and that wax buildup is not a problem. You will sit in a quiet sound booth wearing earphones for most of the testing.

Air Conduction Audiometry

The most basic test is to evaluate your hearing thresholds with pure tones at different frequencies. Like keys on a piano keyboard, the frequencies range from low (on the left of the keyboard) to high (on the right). The threshold is the softest sound you can hear at each frequency. Each ear is tested separately, and this results in an audiogram with the thresholds plotted for each test frequency.

For TRT it is recommended that extra-high frequencies be tested (up to 12,000 Hz).[5] (Hz is the abbreviation for hertz, which refers to cycles per second.) Sometimes hearing loss can be detected in the extra-high frequencies when hearing thresholds are normal in the conventional frequency range (250 Hz to 8,000 Hz). Tinnitus is usually associated with some degree of cochlear impairment, which may not be detected if testing is limited to the conventional frequency range.[131] Studies have shown that hearing loss in the extra-high frequencies may be an early indicator of hearing loss in the conventional range.[132]

Presenting tones through earphones to test hearing thresholds is referred to as *air conduction audiometry* (the sound wave travels through the air from the earphone to the eardrum). With air conduction audiometry, sound waves need to vibrate the eardrum, which vibrates the tiny bones (ossicles) connected to the eardrum (the hammer, anvil, and stirrup—the tiniest bones in the body). The stirrup bone (technically the stapes) connects to the inner ear (the cochlea), where it works like a little piston to transfer the vibrations to the fluid in the cochlea. These vibrations activate the hairs (*stereocilia*) that project above the hair cells into the fluid. Thousands of hair cells are lined up in the cochlea, and they are laid out from low frequencies to high frequencies—just like a piano keyboard (see Fig. 7-3).

Bone Conduction Audiometry

Another method of activating hair cells is by bone conduction. With bone conduction, sound vibrations enter the skull and bypass the eardrum and the tiny bones behind the eardrum to directly activate the fluid in the cochlea. *Bone conduction audiometry* is done to ensure the accuracy of hearing thresholds measured with air conduction audiometry. With bone conduction audiometry, the test tones are presented from a *bone vibrator* that is pressed against the skull behind the ear. Bone conduction audiometry is routinely performed following air conduction audiometry. Differences between air conduction and bone conduction thresholds (*air-bone gaps*) can be due to some obstruction in the air conduction path that sound waves normally take to activate the hair cells in the inner ear. Air-bone gaps could indicate *conductive hearing loss.*

Speech Audiometry

Other tests done by the audiologist involve the use of speech as the test signal that is presented to the patient. The testing is done to estimate how well speech is detected and understood. Most simply, the testing determines *speech reception thresholds* and *speech discrimination scores*. The speech reception threshold (also known as the speech recognition threshold) is the minimum volume level of speech at which a person can understand half (50%) of the words that are presented. To test for speech discrimination, words are presented at a comfortable level and the person repeats them back. The testing can be made more difficult by either reducing the level at which the words are presented or adding background noise to the words.

Loudness Discomfort Levels

An audiometric test that is important for TRT is loudness discomfort levels (LDLs) obtained at the same test frequencies that were used for air conduction audiometry. Results of LDL testing are of "fundamental importance" to assist in determining whether the person has a loudness tolerance problem.[4] A loudness tolerance problem is usually some combination of hyperacusis (physical discomfort to sounds that are comfortable for most people) and misophonia (negative emotions generated by certain sounds). "Almost all patients with hyperacusis have some degree of misophonia."[4 (p. 69)]

For TRT, a specific protocol is recommended for testing LDLs, including the starting level for the test tones, the intensity steps between tone presentations, the rate of testing, and instructions given to patients for how to respond to the testing.[4] LDLs are obtained for each frequency in each ear, and then they are all repeated. Some patients are not comfortable with LDL testing, and if so, they are not required to complete it.

Otoacoustic Emissions

Otoacoustic emissions (OAEs) are sounds that are generated from within the cochlea. More specifically, they are very quiet sounds emitted by the outer hair cells when they vibrate in response to being stimulated by external sound.

With normal hearing, OAEs are present. It doesn't take much hearing loss, however, before OAEs are no longer produced.

Different types of tests can be used to measure for OAEs. One of them is *distortion-product* OAEs (DPOAEs). For TRT, DPOAE testing is considered "useful but not necessary."[4] The DPOAE testing should follow a specific protocol for TRT, and the results can be useful for counseling purposes.

Tinnitus Measures

Additional audiological testing includes tinnitus loudness and pitch matching, as well as minimum masking level (referred to as *minimal suppression level* for TRT). These measures, however, have no direct bearing on the management of tinnitus, and the testing can involve "any generally accepted method."[4]

Summary

The following quote summarizes what is necessary for an audiological evaluation to prepare for TRT: "The following audiological tests are crucial: Loudness discomfort level (LDL), for hyperacusis, and a pure-tone audiogram plus speech discrimination, for hearing loss. Note that these audiological tests alone are not sufficient for making the diagnosis; a detailed interview is essential, particularly to discriminate hyperacusis from misophonia. However, these tests, together with the Initial Interview, are sufficient for diagnosis and proceeding with TRT."[4] (p. 72)

APPENDIX D

Evaluation and Treatment for Decreased Sound Tolerance

It has been estimated that 25 to 30% of people with bothersome tinnitus also have decreased sound tolerance to the extent that treatment would be warranted.[4] For TRT, completing the Initial Interview (chapter 5) and measuring loudness discomfort levels (appendix C) determine whether patients have a significant problem with decreased sound tolerance.

Decreased sound tolerance refers most generally to difficulty tolerating sounds that are comfortable for most other people. A sound tolerance problem usually consists of a combination of hyperacusis and misophonia. The defining feature of category 3 patients is that they are diagnosed with hyperacusis.

Hyperacusis

According to the neurophysiological model (chapter 8), hyperacusis is defined by hypersensitivity to sound that is caused by abnormally strong reactions to sound within the central auditory system. With hyperacusis, the same level of neuronal activity that would normally be evoked by much louder sounds is evoked by softer sounds (for example, neuronal activity evoked by 80 decibels sound pressure level—80 dB SPL—in a person with hyperacusis might be similar to activity evoked by 120 dB SPL in an individual with normal loudness tolerance).

Sounds that cause abnormally strong reactions in the central auditory system can be soft or loud. The reactions are specific to the intensity of the sound as well as its spectral characteristics (its quality or timbre). Any sounds reaching a certain intensity and with similar spectra would consistently cause these reactions. This high level of neuronal activity in the central auditory system causes subsequent activation of the limbic and autonomic nervous systems.

Misophonia

Unlike hyperacusis, misophonia is an *emotional* response to sound. Hyperacusis causes predictable *physical* reactions that are determined by the intensity and spectrum of the offending sound. Misophonic reactions generally have nothing to do with the sound's acoustic characteristics. Rather, according to the neurophysiological model, the central auditory system responds normally to sounds that evoke a misophonic response, but neural connections between the auditory system and the limbic system are enhanced, resulting in strong activation of the limbic and autonomic nervous systems.

Misophonic reactions are *conditioned emotional responses*, meaning they depend on negative memories that are evoked when hearing sounds associated with negative experiences. In essence, misophonia is an aversion to certain sounds that is due to conditioned emotional responses.[4]

It can be difficult to clearly distinguish between effects due to hyperacusis and those due to misophonia. Most people with hyperacusis experience some degree of misophonia. It is also possible for some patients to experience only misophonia without hyperacusis. For example, in a group of 149 tinnitus patients who also had a sound tolerance problem, almost 60% experienced misophonia without a significant hyperacusis problem.[133]

Misophonic patients usually report that they routinely use earplugs and/or earmuffs to prevent exposure to sounds that trigger their emotional reactions. They anticipate these reactions and typically overprotect their ears. The condition can become progressively worse because overprotection causes enhanced sensitivity.[37] The concept of overprotection is important and is explained in chapter 5 (see Initial Interview question 9). Also see question 23 below.

Phonophobia

When fear of sound is a major component of a person's sound tolerance problem, that person is said to have *phonophobia*, which is a subtype of misophonia. The fear is due to *irrational* concerns that certain sounds will (a) worsen the tinnitus, (b) cause physical pain, and/or (c) damage the auditory system. If such concerns are *rational*, however, then the patient is *not* labeled phonophobic. For example, TRT category 4 patients (chapter 3 and appendix E) have rational concerns that their tinnitus and/or hyperacusis is actually worsened by exposure to certain sounds. Some patients, especially those with hyperacusis, experience physical pain when exposed to certain sounds. All people should be concerned about the potential for sound to cause damage to the auditory system if it reaches a certain level of intensity.

Category 3 Placement

It is important that hyperacusis is not confused with misophonia or phonophobia.[4] Of the three conditions, only patients with *significant* hyperacusis (requiring treatment) are placed in TRT category 3. The presence of misophonia or phonophobia does not affect category placement—patients with misophonia or phonophobia can be placed in any category depending on various factors.

Category 3 Treatment

Treatment for hyperacusis (described in further detail below) relies primarily on desensitization through the use of ear-level sound generators set at a comfortable level (the mixing point is irrelevant for treating hyperacusis). Use of sound generators to treat hyperacusis should be continuous during all waking hours. During sleep time some kind of bedside sound generator should be used all night long.

Category 3 patients who require hearing aids will very likely have trouble tolerating amplified sound—especially early in treatment. Most current hearing aids are combination instruments (hearing aid combined with sound generator in one shell), which are optimal for these patients. The strategy is to first use the sound generators with very low amplification and high compression (which limits the maximum amplification of sound to keep it within a comfortable range). Alternatively, only the sound generators can be used as the first stage of treatment to start the desensitization process. With sufficient desensitization, amplification can be added and gradually increased over time as appropriate.

It is important to determine whether the patient has hyperacusis, misophonia, or both. The protocols for treating hyperacusis and misophonia are distinctly different. Also, if hyperacusis is a significant problem in an individual with bothersome tinnitus, it should be the main focus of treatment. If misophonia is a significant problem, it can be treated concurrently with tinnitus.

Initial Interview

In chapter 5, we went through the TRT Initial Interview question by question. The Interview contains three sections: Tinnitus, Sound Tolerance, and Hearing. We completed the questions from the Tinnitus section and the Hearing section, and we only asked the first question (question 19) from the Sound Tolerance section. Because sound tolerance was not a problem for our hypothetical patient, we skipped questions 20 through 30 from the Sound Tolerance section. We will now cover those questions, starting with a "yes" response to question 19.

Question 19. Are sounds bothersome or unpleasant to you when they seem normal to other people around you? *If yes*, what kinds of sounds are bothersome or unpleasant?

If patients answer "yes," then they are asked to indicate the kinds of sounds that cause the problem. A list of different categories of sounds is provided below. It is suggested that, without looking at the list, you write down the kinds of sounds that you find bothersome or unpleasant. Then look at the list and see which kinds of sounds would correspond with what you wrote down.

☐ **Higher-pitched sounds** (*examples*: squeals, squeaks, beeps, whistles, rings)

☐ **Lower-pitched sounds** (*examples*: bass from radio, next door music)

☐ **Traffic (warning) sounds** (*examples*: emergency vehicle sirens, car horns, back-up beeper on truck/van)

☐ **Traffic (background) sounds** (*examples*: road noise, road construction, diesel engines, garbage trucks)

☐ **Sudden impact sounds** (*examples*: door slam, car back-firing, objects dropping on floor, dishes clattering)

☐ **Voices** (*examples*: television, radio, movies, children's voices, dog barking)

☐ **Other** (describe) _____

Question 20. Do these sounds cause you pain or physical discomfort?

Hypersensitivity to sound can involve hyperacusis, misophonia, and phonophobia. Before you answer this question, let's review the definitions for each of these conditions directly from the Jastreboff and Hazell (2004) book:

Hyperacusis

"Abnormally strong reaction to sound occurring within the auditory pathways. At the behavioral level, it is manifested by a patient experiencing physical discomfort as a result of exposure to sound (quiet, medium, or loud). The same sound would not evoke a similar reaction in an average listener. The strength of the reaction is controlled by the physical characteristics of the sound (e.g., its spectrum and intensity). It can result from both peripheral and central auditory dysfunction."[4] (Glossary)

Misophonia

"Abnormally strong reactions of the autonomic and limbic systems resulting from enhanced connections between the auditory and limbic systems. Importantly, misophonia and phonophobia do not involve significant activation of the auditory system."[4] (Glossary)

Phonophobia

"A specific form of misophonia when fear of sound is the dominant emotion."[4] (Glossary)

Distinguishing between these three conditions helps to clarify which components are involved in the sound tolerance problem. While there may be subtle differences between the conditions, it is important to make the correct diagnosis because treatment will differ depending on the specific condition.[7]

Question 20 specifically addresses hyperacusis, which can briefly be described as a *physiological (not psychological) response to sound involving some level of physical discomfort.* People with significant hyperacusis almost always also have misophonia, especially those who have had long-term hyperacusis.[4,133]

Question 21. Do you have "bad days" when sound tolerance is more of a problem than on other days, or is your ability to tolerate sound the same from day to day? *If yes*, how often do you have these bad days?

Question 21 is the same as question 7 from the Initial Interview, except that it is specific to a sound tolerance problem rather than to tinnitus. People generally know if their sound tolerance problem is more bothersome on some days than on others. If they answer *yes*, then they are asked to estimate how often these bad days occur (number of days per week, month, or year). Their responses to this question over the period of treatment are helpful in determining how well the treatment is working to reduce their sound tolerance problem.

Question 22. Do sounds ever cause a change in how much sound you can tolerate? *If less able to tolerate sound*, what kinds of sounds cause a change in your ability to tolerate sound? When any of these sounds reduce your sound tolerance, how long does the change last? When you hear a sound that reduces your ability to tolerate sounds, does the effect sometimes last until the next morning after you've slept? *If yes*, what kinds of sounds cause this to happen?

Question 22 is similar to question 8 from the Initial Interview. Whereas question 8 was specific to tinnitus, question 22 is specific to sound tolerance. Certain exposures to sound can worsen a tinnitus problem and can also worsen a sound tolerance problem. Question 22 helps to determine whether a person should be appropriately placed in TRT category 4, indicating that exposure to certain sounds causes prolonged worsening of sound sensitivity until at least the next morning. Category 4 thus pertains to both tinnitus and hyperacusis, and some people have prolonged worsening to both conditions simultaneously. Successful outcome of treatment is less assured for category 4 patients than for the other categories, and extended treatment may be necessary.

Question 22 is actually a series of questions to obtain all of the information necessary to determine whether category 4 placement is appropriate. The series of questions is essentially the same as for question 8 from the Initial Interview (see question 8 in chapter 5 for further explanation). When asking this question in-person with patients, clinicians are advised to not mention the types of sounds that are listed in the Interview (see below). The idea is that if patients volunteer this information without being prompted, the most relevant responses are obtained. You as the reader can think about how you would answer these questions and then look at the list below and see which types of sounds might pertain to your personal experiences.

- ☐ **Very loud sounds/activities** (*examples*: firing a gun, attending a concert, using power tools)

- ☐ **Higher-pitched sounds** (*examples*: squeals, squeaks, beeps, whistles, rings)

- ☐ **Lower-pitched sounds** (*examples*: bass from radio, next door music)

- ☐ **Traffic (warning) sounds** (*examples*: emergency vehicle sirens, car horns, back-up beeper on truck/van)

- ☐ **Traffic (background) sounds** (*examples*: road noise, road construction, diesel engines, garbage trucks)

- ☐ **Sudden impact sounds** (*examples*: door slam, car backfiring, objects dropping on floor, dishes clattering)

- ☐ **Voices** (*examples*: television, radio, movies, children's voices, dog barking)

- ☐ **Other** (describe) _____

Question 23. (<u>Interviewer</u>: In Question 9 did the patient report the use of hearing protection because of "trouble tolerating everyday sounds"?) *If yes:* **Earlier you told me that you sometimes use ear protection because of trouble tolerating sound— what percent of the time do you use ear protection** *because of that trouble?* **Do you use your earplugs when it's fairly quiet** *because of trouble tolerating sound?* **(<u>Interviewer</u>: Does patient** *overprotect* **ears** *due to problems with sound tolerance?***)**

Question 9 from the Initial Interview asks if hearing protection is used because of "trouble tolerating everyday sounds that seem normal to others." If the response to this question was *no*, then question 23 can be skipped. If the response was *yes*, then the follow-up questions are asked. The purpose of question 9 is to determine whether people overprotect their ears to prevent their tinnitus from becoming worse. Similarly, the purpose of question 23 is to determine whether there is overuse of hearing protection because of worries that sound will worsen a sound sensitivity problem. If this is determined to be the case, it is essential to address the concern that *overuse of hearing protection can increase sensitivity to sound.*[134]

Question 24. Are you currently receiving any treatment specifically for problems with *sound tolerance*? If yes, what?

Although it is less likely that someone would be receiving treatment for a sound tolerance problem than for a tinnitus problem, it is important to rule out this possibility. It would be counterproductive to receive or to self-administer any kind of therapy that could worsen hyperacusis or otherwise conflict with TRT. If sound is already being used for desensitization purposes, that should be pointed out as appropriate as long as its use is consistent with TRT sound therapy.

Question 25. What is the major reason *trouble tolerating sound* is a problem?

This should be the definitive question to identify the primary objective of treatment. The question is asked before the follow-up question (26) that provides a list of potential reasons why sound tolerance is a problem. Asking question 25 as an open-ended question should reveal the most bothersome aspect of hyperacusis that should be addressed with treatment. Question 26 then suggests numerous possibilities as to what might also be affected by the sound tolerance problem.

> **Question 26. I'm going to read through a list of activities, and I want you to tell me how often trouble tolerating sound keeps you from doing these activities, or how often it negatively affects these activities in any way. Please don't include trouble hearing or trouble understanding speech when you answer these questions.**

Like question 12 from the Initial Interview that addresses how tinnitus affects life activities, question 26 provides a list of activities that may be affected by the sound tolerance problem. The activities listed for questions 12 and 26 are somewhat different because life activities are affected differently by tinnitus compared to sound tolerance problems.

After each activity, response options are *never, rarely, sometimes, often,* or *always* (or *N/A*). A response profile is then created, showing those activities that are the most affected. The most successful outcome of treatment would be seen if all responses were "rarely" or "never."

	Never	Rarely	Some-times	Often	Always	N/A
Concerts?	☐	☐	☐	☐	☐	☐
Shopping?	☐	☐	☐	☐	☐	☐
Movies?	☐	☐	☐	☐	☐	☐
Work? (select NIA if retired)	☐	☐	☐	☐	☐	☐

	Never	Rarely	Some-times	Often	Always	N/A
Day-to-day responsibilities outside of work?	☐	☐	☐	☐	☐	☐
Going to restaurants?	☐	☐	☐	☐	☐	☐
Driving?	☐	☐	☐	☐	☐	☐
Participating in or observing sports events?	☐	☐	☐	☐	☐	☐
Attending church?	☐	☐	☐	☐	☐	☐
Housekeeping activities?	☐	☐	☐	☐	☐	☐
Child care?	☐	☐	☐	☐	☐	☐
Social activities?	☐	☐	☐	☐	☐	☐
Anything else?	☐	☐	☐	☐	☐	☐

I'm now going to ask you to *rank* your sound tolerance, on a scale of 0 to 10, with regard to its severity, annoyance, and effect on your life.

Question 27. Please rate your ability to tolerate sound on a scale of 0 to 10. "0" would mean "you can tolerate all sounds"; "10" would mean "you cannot tolerate any sounds."

Can tolerate all   0 1 2 3 4 5 6 7 8 9 10   Can't tolerate any

Question 28. How much has trouble tolerating sound *annoyed you*, on average, over the last month? "0" would be "not annoying at all"; "10" would be "as annoying as you can imagine."

| Can tolerate all | 0 | 1 | 2 | 3 | 4 | 5 | 6 | 7 | 8 | 9 | 10 | Can't tolerate any |

Question 29. How much did trouble tolerating sound affect your life, on average, over the last month? "0" would be "not at all"; "10" would be "as much as you can imagine."

| Can tolerate all | 0 | 1 | 2 | 3 | 4 | 5 | 6 | 7 | 8 | 9 | 10 | Can't tolerate any |

Questions 27, 28, and 29 each address a different perspective on how decreased sound tolerance can be a problem. For each question, a number is selected between 0 and 10 to best represent the degree of difficulty caused by the sound tolerance problem. It would be expected for most people that the response numbers would be similar across the three questions.

Question 30. Do you have any other comments about *trouble tolerating sound*?

Question 30 is the final question in the Sound Tolerance section of the Initial Interview. It gives the person one more opportunity to express any thoughts about the sound tolerance problem that has been addressed throughout this section. By this point it should be clear whether the problem is hyperacusis, misophonia, phonophobia, or some combination of these conditions. It needs to be clear what the problem is to know how to best prescribe the approach to treatment.

Follow-up Interview

The questions in the Sound Tolerance section of the Follow-up Interview should be answered only if decreased sound tolerance was listed as a problem on the Initial Interview. If sound tolerance was not considered a problem prior to treatment, then it will very likely not be a problem at later visits. Because of exceptions, however, it is important to at least ask if sound tolerance is a problem during treatment. If sound tolerance was reported as a problem prior to treatment, then all of the questions in the Sound Tolerance section of the Follow-up Interview should be answered.

In the Follow-up Interview, the questions in the Sound Tolerance section (questions 13 through 22) are almost identical to those in the Sound Tolerance section (questions 19 through 30) in the Initial Interview. The only significant difference between Interview versions is that question 14 in the Follow-up Interview asks if the number of "bad days" caused by decreased sound tolerance has changed (Do you have these bad days "more often," "less often," or "just as often" as before you started treatment? Are your bad days "the same," "not as bad," or "worse" than before you started treatment?).

When asking the sound tolerance questions in the Follow-up Interview, it is important to compare these responses to the corresponding responses from the Initial Interview. When comparing between versions, people are often surprised at how much progress has been made.

Questions 24–26 on the Follow-up Interview are asked to assess the *impact* (on a scale of 0 to 10) of tinnitus (question 24: How much of a problem is *tinnitus?*), decreased sound tolerance (question 25: How much of a problem is *trouble tolerating sound?*), and hearing loss (question 26: How much of a problem is *hearing?*) on the person's life. If more than one of these conditions is a significant problem, it is important at every visit to determine which condition is thought to have the greatest impact. These *relative rankings* can change during treatment. For example, significant hearing loss would be treated with hearing aids, which should result in hearing becoming much less of a problem. Or, if someone has both tinnitus and hyperacusis, and hyperacusis is the main problem, then it is treated first. Once the hyperacusis problem is sufficiently resolved, then the tinnitus becomes the focus of treatment.

Counseling for Decreased Sound Tolerance

Counseling for hyperacusis always starts by covering the structured TRT counseling from its beginning through the Auditory Gain section (see chapter 7). Most people with hyperacusis also have some degree of misophonia, so the counseling usually addresses both of these concerns.

With respect to the neurophysiological model, misophonia involves the same neural connections as for bothersome tinnitus—the limbic system is activated in both instances. It is therefore important to understand the neurophysiological model from the perspective of *annoying sound* triggering reactions rather than tinnitus.

Counseling for both hyperacusis and misophonia should include all of Topic 5 (Plasticity of the Brain—chapter 7) and relevant portions of Topic 6 (The Neurophysiological Model of Tinnitus—chapter 8).

Like the tinnitus counseling that is provided word for word in chapters 7 and 8, counseling for hyperacusis is provided in the sections below. The script is based directly on the counseling protocol described by Jastreboff and Hazell[4] (Section 3.4.2; pp. 106-108) and emphasizes possible neural mechanisms underlying the condition.

A resource to supplement the sound tolerance counseling is the book *Tinnitus Retraining Therapy: Patient Counseling Guide*.[10] The counseling corresponds with Section 8 (Hyperacusis) in that book. Pictures and graphics are provided for each counseling topic, which can be helpful for understanding the concepts being taught.

Counseling for Hyperacusis

It is first essential to clearly understand the differences between hyperacusis, misophonia, and phonophobia. This would be a good time to review their definitions provided above for question 20 from the Initial Interview.

Automatic Gain Control

The auditory system has automatic gain control, a concept I have explained in detail elsewhere.[3,22,41] Briefly, automatic gain control means that the auditory system automatically adjusts its sensitivity to sound according to the intensity of sound that is experienced. The general rule for auditory gain is: as sound becomes *louder*, gain *decreases*; as sound becomes *softer*, gain *increases*.[3] This is a principle that's critical to understand with respect to treatment for hyperacusis.

A study was completed that perfectly depicts how sound and auditory gain are related in real life.[37] This research group compared the effects of *adding* versus *reducing* sound to the ears. The added-sound group of participants wore ear-level sound generators for two weeks. The reduced-sound group wore earplugs for two weeks. Sensitivity to sound was measured before and after the two weeks. What do you think was the result?

The added-sound group had reduced sensitivity to sound (equating to greater tolerance of sound). The "volume control" in their brain was turned down (auditory gain was reduced), which gave them greater ability to tolerate the loudness of sounds.

The reduced-sound group had greater sensitivity to sound (equating to reduced tolerance). Their "volume control" was turned up (auditory gain was increased), resulting in reduced ability to tolerate the loudness of sounds.

Here is a simple way to think about the relationship between exposure to sound and the ability to tolerate the loudness of sound:

- ↑ **sound** → ↓ auditory gain → ↑ **tolerance** to the loudness of sound
- ↓ **sound** → ↑ auditory gain → ↓ **tolerance** to the loudness of sound

These adjustments to loudness sensitivity take place both in the cochlea and in the central auditory pathways. When we hear very soft sounds, those sounds can be amplified by as much as 60 decibels (dB) by the outer hair cells. (Please review Hair Cell Loss: Outer versus Inner in chapter 7.) Further amplification can take place in the central auditory pathways. As the level of sound increases, the amplification (auditory gain) decreases accordingly (↑ sound → ↓ auditory gain).

Hyperacusis

If the auditory gain mechanism provides too much amplification, sounds can seem abnormally loud. For the person with hyperacusis, sounds that are easily tolerated by most people become uncomfortably loud, or even painful.

A sound tolerance condition that is limited to hyperacusis (*pure hyperacusis*) primarily involves increased gain in the auditory pathways. This overamplification causes activation of the limbic and autonomic nervous systems.

Testing Loudness Discomfort Levels

Testing for hyperacusis involves measuring loudness discomfort levels (see appendix C) and conducting a detailed interview, which we covered earlier in this appendix. To measure loudness discomfort levels, pure tones delivered from an audiometer are made increasingly louder until they reach a level that is uncomfortably loud. If you have normal loudness tolerance, your loudness discomfort levels will be around 100 decibels Hearing Level (100 dB HL) or higher, and those numbers can be plotted on your audiogram (which shows your hearing thresholds in dB HL). With hyperacusis, loudness discomfort levels are reduced below 100 dB HL— often substantially reduced (such as down to 60 or 70 dB HL).

It should be noted that testing loudness discomfort levels can be an uncomfortable experience for some people. This testing should therefore be done with extreme caution and postponed or avoided in some circumstances.

Treating Hyperacusis

The underlying problem with hyperacusis is hypersensitivity of the auditory system to sound (too much gain). The objective of treating hyperacusis is to reverse the hypersensitivity by *desensitizing* the auditory system to sound (by decreasing the gain, or "turning down the volume"—just like the added-sound group in the experiment we discussed above).

Desensitizing the auditory system is accomplished by systematic exposure to sounds that cause absolutely no annoyance or discomfort. This procedure generally results in a gradual increase in the ability to listen comfortably to sounds that are progressively louder. When this desensitization procedure is successful, testing for loudness discomfort levels will show an increase in how much sound a person can tolerate comfortably. Increased loudness tolerance can be observed in as little as a few weeks.

Counseling for Misophonia

Most people with hyperacusis also have misophonia. Whereas hyperacusis is caused by overamplification in the auditory system, misophonia results from activation of the limbic and autonomic nervous systems whenever a sound causes discomfort.

The emotional and autonomic (stress) reactions to sounds that define misophonia result from conditioned reflexes. The brain learns (becomes conditioned) to interpret certain sounds as uncomfortable or annoying because they are associated with negative memories. Evoking those memories with certain sounds triggers emotional and stress reactions.

With respect to the neurophysiological model (chapter 8), misophonia involves the same connections in the brain as for a tinnitus problem. These connections are between the auditory, limbic, and autonomic nervous systems.

Treatment of Misophonia

To treat hyperacusis, the objective is to reduce gain in the auditory system, which enables tolerance to higher levels of sound. Treatment of misophonia uses a different approach. With misophonia, the connections between the auditory, limbic, and autonomic nervous systems that cause the emotional reactions must be retrained. This retraining is accomplished when the conditioned reflexes responsible for these reactions are extinguished.

Extinguishing the conditioned reflexes that underlie misophonia requires consistently creating *positive associations with sound*. The typical treatment is to be exposed to pleasant sound while paying attention to it. The key is to *listen* to pleasant sounds, which is the opposite of what is recommended for hyperacusis. With hyperacusis, sounds need to be neutral, in the background, and mostly ignored. With misophonia, *active listening* to enjoyable sounds results in positive feelings about listening to sound in general, which eventually extinguishes the conditioned reflexes.

As already mentioned, hyperacusis and misophonia usually occur together. Treatment therefore should include both desensitization of the auditory system to address the hyperacusis and active listening to pleasant sounds to address the misophonia.

Counseling for Phonophobia

Misophonia refers to emotional reactions to sound. Phonophobia is a subtype of misophonia involving *fear of sound*. If a person's reactions to sound do *not* involve fear, then the condition is not phonophobia.

People with tinnitus or hyperacusis may become fearful that certain sounds will damage the auditory system or worsen their tinnitus and/or hyperacusis. Because of this fear, they may overprotect their ears by using hearing protection (earplugs or earmuffs) or avoiding sound altogether. What they don't realize is that the sounds they fear are generally harmless.

Overprotecting the ears by blocking or avoiding sound can make the auditory system even more sensitive, which actually worsens the sound tolerance condition. We previously discussed the study with the added-sound and reduced-sound groups.[37] The group that wore earplugs (reduced sound) became more sensitive to sound, which demonstrated how overprotecting the ears can worsen a sound tolerance problem.

Treatment for phonophobia involves counseling that specifically addresses the benign nature of sounds that cause the phonophobic reaction and that the auditory system needs to be exposed to such sounds to maintain normal functioning. In addition, the same sound therapy protocol that is used for misophonia is used for phonophobia.

Ongoing Treatment

Successful treatment for hyperacusis usually starts to be observed within a few weeks, and full resolution can occur within some number of months. Some people eventually achieve a total cure for their hyperacusis and/or misophonia. The time period for noticing improvement depends on many factors.

Importantly, treatment for hyperacusis should occur on a different schedule than for tinnitus. The hyperacusis treatment schedule depends mainly on the severity of the problem. Anyone with very severe hyperacusis should visit with the TRT clinician every week. Those with more moderate severity might need visits every two to three weeks. These intervals are maintained for only as long as necessary to achieve sufficient improvement.

When hyperacusis is under control, treatment should shift to addressing the tinnitus problem (which is the case for most people with a moderate to severe hyperacusis problem). With misophonia, the treatment schedule generally follows the protocol used with TRT category 1 and 2 patients, as described in chapter 9.

We've discussed testing for loudness discomfort levels (in this appendix and in appendix C). Determining the effects of treatment for hyperacusis involves retesting loudness discomfort levels and administering the TRT Follow-up Interview (described earlier in this appendix). These evaluations should be done at every visit. Retesting loudness discomfort levels can help to document any reported change in sound tolerance that might be noted on the Follow-up Interview. Obtaining loudness discomfort levels also assists in determining the level of sound that can be used for treatment.[4]

As already noted, measuring loudness discomfort levels can be uncomfortable for some people. The testing should not be done if it has this effect. Otherwise, the testing should always be done with extreme caution and possibly postponed or avoided depending on how the person feels about it.

APPENDIX E

Evaluation and Treatment for Category 4

For some people, exposure to certain sounds can cause their tinnitus to become more intense and/or reduce their ability to tolerate sound (if they have hyperacusis). As explained in chapter 3, the defining feature of TRT category 4 patients is that such worsening of either or both of these conditions lasts until at least the next day. The effect can actually last for days or even weeks. It is essential for category 4 patients to receive appropriate treatment "because inappropriate treatment can have devastating results."4 (p. 131)

For most people in category 4, hyperacusis is the dominant problem and the counseling described in appendix D should be completed.4 Aside from the counseling, the primary objective is to desensitize the auditory pathways using continuous sound. The sound should be presented at the highest comfortable level above threshold (which is usually very low) without producing winding-up or kindling effects. (*Winding-up* refers to tinnitus and/or hyperacusis being worsened for an extended period due to exposure to some continuous sound. *Kindling* refers to a situation when exposure to sound initially causes no discomfort but starts to evoke discomfort after several exposures.)

People with strong misophonia can have symptoms that would seemingly qualify them for placement in category 4.[4] *Strong misophonia* would be described as relatively severe emotional reactions to sound that carry over until the next day. It is therefore important to distinguish strong misophonia from the prolonged worsening of tinnitus and/or hyperacusis due to sound exposure that defines category 4.

A history of Lyme disease, head injury, or neurological problems would make a person more likely to be assigned to category 4.[4] Regardless of any disease or condition that might be associated with the symptoms that define category 4, the primary aim of treatment is to desensitize the auditory system in the same manner as for treatment of hyperacusis. Because of possible extreme sensitivity to sound, it may be necessary to use sound at near-threshold levels to start the desensitization process. Using sound at near-threshold levels raises concerns about inducing stochastic resonance (explained in chapter 6). This is a secondary concern, but people should at least be aware of it. They should also stay alert to how sound might cause different effects depending on its level relative to the threshold of hearing. The most conservative method for using sound, with the least risk of worsening tinnitus or hyperacusis, is to start at a level just above threshold and very gradually increase the level over time.

The standard sound therapy protocol for category 4 is to wear ear-level sound generators (or hearing aids with a built-in sound generator) and adjust the sound output to a low and comfortable level for the first few weeks.[4] Some people experience *global hypersensitivity*, meaning they are also hypersensitive to touch. They may need a week or more just to get used to the feel of the devices on their ears, which can be accomplished by wearing the devices without switching on the sound generator. Treatment would then progress in blocks of six to eight weeks, with each block involving a slight increase in the level of sound presented from the sound generators. If the tinnitus or hyperacusis worsens during any one block, then the level would be reduced to what was comfortable during the previous block. It is always essential to use the sound generators continuously throughout each day.

As already mentioned, category 4 is the most difficult of all the TRT categories to successfully treat. Also, even with positive results, recovery generally takes longer than for the other categories. Further information about treatment for this challenging and unpredictable category can be found in the definitive TRT book.[4] (especially pp. 131-133)

About the Author

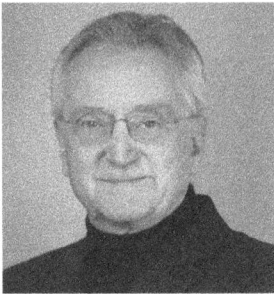

James A. Henry, PhD, is an audiologist with a doctorate in behavioral neuroscience. His six years working on his doctorate under the tutelage of Drs. Mary Meikle and Jack Vernon ignited his passionate interest in tinnitus research. During his career of over 35 years, he received funding of $28 million as principal or co-principal investigator for 43 projects and grants. He has authored 240 articles, including 135 in peer-reviewed journals and six books about tinnitus. He gave lectures and presentations nationally and internationally. His accomplishments resulted in numerous awards, including the Veterans Affairs (VA) Rehabilitation Research and Development 2016 Paul B. Magnuson Award *("the highest honor for VA rehabilitation investigators")* and the Jerger Career Award for Research in Audiology from the American Academy of Audiology Honors Committee.

Dr. Henry, who retired in September 2022, continues to give lectures and training workshops, serves as a consultant, and has maintained his role as editor-at-large for the American Tinnitus Association's journal *Tinnitus Today*. His primary interest, however, is writing books about tinnitus, hyperacusis, and hearing loss. This book is the second in a series of books he has planned under his corporation Ears Gone Wrong, LLC. These books are intended for the general public to be easily understood with practical information for addressing auditory problems.

His website is www.earsgonewrong.org

Acknowledgments

This book is dedicated to Pawel J. Jastreboff, PhD, ScD, MBA—the founder of TRT. I am indebted to Dr. Jastreboff for providing me with TRT training in the 1990s and for his support of my research projects, books, and articles about TRT.

Certain individuals made significant contributions to the development and refining of TRT. They include Margaret Jastreboff, Jonathan W.P. Hazell, Jacqueline Sheldrake, Susan Gold, and Craig Formby. Additionally, many others have contributed since those early days.

This book received significant edits by my supportive wife, Mary Jo. The book was also edited by Stephen M. Nagler, MD who made many important contributions. It was professionally proofread and copyedited by Robin L. Reed.

The overall contents of this book are the direct result of my 35-year research career. Dozens of colleagues and acquaintances have informed my thinking about tinnitus. I thank each and every one of them.

References

1.   Henry JA, Manning C. Clinical pro-
     tocol to promote standardization of basic
     tinnitus services by audiologists. *Amer-
     ican Journal of Audiology*. 2019;28(1S):152-161.
     doi:10.1044/2018_AJA-TTR17-18-0038

2.   Langguth B, Kleinjung T, Landgrebe M. Tinnitus:
     the complexity of standardization. *Evalua-
     tion and the Health Professions*. 2011;34(4):429-33.
     doi:10.1177/0163278710394337

3.   Henry JA. *The Tinnitus Book: Understanding Tinnitus
     and How To Find Relief*. Ears Gone Wrong, LLC. 2023.

4.   Jastreboff PJ, Hazell JWP. *Tinnitus Retraining Therapy:
     Implementing the Neurophysiological Model*. Cambridge
     University Press; 2004.

5.   Jastreboff PJ. Tinnitus Retraining Therapy. In: Moller
     AR, Langguth B, DeRidder D, Kleinjung T, eds. *Text-
     book of Tinnitus*. Springer; 2011:575-596.

6. Jastreboff PJ. Tinnitus Habituation Therapy (THT) and Tinnitus Retraining Therapy (TRT). In: Tyler R, ed. *Tinnitus Handbook*. Singular Publishing Group; 2000:357-376.

7. Jastreboff PJ, Jastreboff MM. Tinnitus Retraining Therapy (TRT) as a method for treatment of tinnitus and hyperacusis patients. *Journal of the American Academy of Audiology*. 2000;11(3):162-77.

8. Jastreboff PJ, Jastreboff MM. Tinnitus Retraining Therapy. *Seminars in Hearing*. 2001;22:51-63.

9. Henry JA, Jastreboff MM, Jastreboff PJ, Schechter MA, Fausti SA. Assessment of patients for treatment with Tinnitus Retraining Therapy. *Journal of the American Academy of Audiology*. 2002;13(10):523-44.

10. Henry JA, Trune DR, Robb MJA, Jastreboff PJ. *Tinnitus Retraining Therapy: Patient Counseling Guide*. Plural Publishing, Inc.; 2007.

11. Henry JA, Jastreboff MM, Jastreboff PJ, Schechter MA, Fausti SA. Guide to conducting Tinnitus Retraining Therapy initial and follow-up interviews. *Journal of Rehabilitative Research and Development*. 2003;40(2):157-77.

12. Fuller TE, Haider HF, Kikidis D, et al. Different teams, same conclusions? A systematic review of existing clinical guidelines for the assessment and treatment of tinnitus in adults. *Frontiers in Psychology*. 2017;8:206. doi:10.3389/fpsyg.2017.00206

13. Cima RFF, Mazurek B, Haider H, et al. A multidisciplinary European guideline for tinnitus: diagnostics, assessment, and treatment. *HNO*. 2019;67(Suppl 1):10-42. doi:10.1007/s00106-019-0633-7

14. Tunkel DE, Bauer CA, Sun GH, et al. Clinical practice guideline: tinnitus. *Otolaryngology Head and Neck Surgery*. 2014;151(2 Suppl):S1-S40. doi:10.1177/0194599814545325

15. Theodoroff SM. Tinnitus questionnaires for research and clinical use. *Current Topics in Behavioral Neuroscience*. 2021;51:403-418. doi:10.1007/7854_2020_175

16. Newman CW, Sandridge SA, Jacobson GP. Assessing outcomes of tinnitus intervention. *Journal of the American Academy of Audiology*. 2014;25(1):76-105. doi:10.3766/jaaa.25.1.6

17. Meikle MB, Henry JA, Griest SE, et al. The Tinnitus Functional Index: development of a new clinical measure for chronic, intrusive tinnitus. *Ear and Hearing*. 2012;33(2):153-76. doi:10.1097/AUD.0b013e31822f67c0

18. Henry JA, Griest S, Thielman E, McMillan G, Kaelin C, Carlson KF. Tinnitus Functional Index: Development, validation, outcomes research, and clinical application. *Hearing Research*. 2016;334:58-64. doi:10.1016/j.heares.2015.06.004

19. Henry JA, Schechter MA, Nagler SM, Fausti SA. Comparison of tinnitus masking and tinnitus retraining therapy. *Journal of the American Academy of Audiology*. 2002;13(10):559-81.

20. Jastreboff PJ. Categories of the patients in TRT and the treatment outcome. In: Hazell JWP, ed. *Proceedings of the Sixth International Tinnitus Seminar 1999.* The Tinnitus and Hyperacusis Centre; 1999:394-398.

21. Jastreboff PJ. Tinnitus. In: Gates GA, ed. *Current Therapy in Otolaryngology–Head and Neck Surgery.* 6th ed. Mosby-YearBook, Inc.; 1998:90-95.

22. Henry JA, Theodoroff SM, Edmonds C, et al. Sound tolerance conditions (hyperacusis, misophonia, noise sensitivity, and phonophobia): definitions and clinical management. *American Journal of Audiology.* 2022;31(3):513-527. doi:10.1044/2022_AJA-22-00035

23. Henry JA, Griest S, Zaugg TL, et al. Tinnitus and Hearing Survey: a screening tool to differentiate bothersome tinnitus from hearing difficulties. *American Journal of Audiology.* 2015;24(1):66-77. doi:10.1044/2014_AJA-14-0042

24. Ratnayake SA, Jayarajan V, Bartlett J. Could an underlying hearing loss be a significant factor in the handicap caused by tinnitus? *Noise and Health.* 2009;11(44):156-60. doi:10.4103/1463-1741.53362

25. Jastreboff MM, Jastreboff PJ. Questionnaires for assessment of the patients and their outcomes. In: Hazell JWP, ed. *Proceedings of the Sixth International Tinnitus Seminar.* The Tinnitus and Hyperacusis Centre; 1999:487-491.

26. Rizan C, Das P, Low R, et al. A streamlined pathway for patients with unilateral tinnitus: Our experience of 22 patients. *Clinical Otolaryngology*. 2019;44(2):191-196. doi:10.1111/coa.13258

27. Abbas Y, Smith G, Trinidade A. Audiologist-led screening of acoustic neuromas in patients with asymmetrical sensorineural hearing loss and/or unilateral tinnitus: our experience in 1126 patients. *Journal of Laryngology and Otology*. 2018;132(9):786-789. doi:10.1017/S0022215118001561

28. Henry JA, Griest S, Austin D, et al. Tinnitus Screener: Results from the first 100 participants in an epidemiology study. *American Journal of Audiology*. 2016;25(2):153-60. doi:10.1044/2016_AJA-15-0076

29. Thielman EJ, Reavis KM, Theodoroff SM, et al. Tinnitus Screener: Short-term test-retest reliability. *American Journal of Audiology*. 2023;32(1):232-242. doi:10.1044/2022_AJA-22-00140

30. Meikle MB. Methods for evaluation of tinnitus relief procedures. In: Aran J-M, Dauman R, eds. *Proceedings IV International Tinnitus Seminar, Bordeaux*. Kugler Publications; 1991:555-562.

31. Meikle M, Taylor-Walsh E. Characteristics of tinnitus and related observations in over 1800 tinnitus clinic patients. *Journal of Laryngology and Otology Supplement*. 1984;9:17-21. doi:10.1017/s1755146300090053

32. Elarbed A, Fackrell K, Baguley DM, Hoare DJ. Tinnitus and stress in adults: a scoping review. *International Journal of Audiology.* 2021;60(3):171-182. doi:10.1080/14992027.2020.1827306

33. Pupic-Bakrac J, Pupic-Bakrac A. Comorbidity of chronic tinnitus and psychological stress - which came first, the chicken or the egg? *Psychiatria Danubia.* 2020;32(Suppl 4):412-419.

34. Unterrainer J, Greimel KV, Leibetseder M, Koller T. Experiencing tinnitus: which factors are important for perceived severity of the symptom? *International Tinnitus Journal.* 2003;9(2):130-3.

35. Andersson G. Tinnitus loudness matchings in relation to annoyance and grading of severity. *Auris Nasus Larynx.* 2003;30(2):129-33. doi:10.1016/s0385-8146(03)00008-7

36. Henry JA. "Measurement" of tinnitus. *Otology and Neurotology.* 2016;37(8):e276-85. doi:10.1097/MAO.0000000000001070

37. Formby C, Sherlock LP, Gold SL. Adaptive plasticity of loudness induced by chronic attenuation and enhancement of the acoustic background. *Journal of the Acoustical Society of America.* 2003;114(1):55-8. doi:10.1121/1.1582860

38. Vidal JL, Park JM, Han JS, Alshaikh H, Park SN. Measurement of loudness discomfort levels as a test for hyperacusis: test-retest reliability and its clinical value. *Clinical and Experimental Otorhinolaryngology.* 2022;15(1):84-90. doi:10.21053/ceo.2021.00318

39. Pienkowski M. Rationale and efficacy of sound therapies for tinnitus and hyperacusis. *Neuroscience*. 2019;407:120-134. doi:10.1016/j.neuroscience.2018.09.012

40. Sheppard A, Stocking C, Ralli M, Salvi R. A review of auditory gain, low-level noise and sound therapy for tinnitus and hyperacusis. *International Journal of Audiology*. 2020;59(1):5-15. doi:10.1080/14992027.2019.1660812

41. Henry JA. Sound therapy to reduce auditory gain for hyperacusis and tinnitus. *American Journal of Audiology*. 2022;31(4):1067-1077. doi:10.1044/2022_AJA-22-00127

42. Henry JA. Directed attention and habituation: two concepts critical to tinnitus management. *American Journal of Audiology*. 2023:1-8. doi:10.1044/2022_AJA-22-00178

43. Henry JA, McMillan L, Manning C. Multidisciplinary tinnitus care. *The Journal for Nurse Practitioners*. 2019;15:671-675.

44. Jastreboff PJ. Clinical implication of the neurophysiological model of tinnitus. In: Reich GE, Vernon JA, eds. *Proceedings of the Fifth International Tinnitus Seminar 1995*. American Tinnitus Association; 1996:500-507.

45. Jastreboff PJ, Gray WC, Gold SL. Neurophysiological approach to tinnitus patients. *American Journal of Otology*. 1996;17(2):236-40.

46. Jastreboff PJ, Hazell JWP. Treatment of tinnitus based on a neurophysiological model. In: Vernon JA, ed. *Tinnitus Treatment and Relief.* Allyn & Bacon; 1998:201-217.

47. Manning C, Grush L, Thielman E, Roberts L, Henry JA. Comparison of tinnitus loudness measures: matching, rating, and scaling. *American Journal of Audiology.* 2019;28(1):137-143. doi:10.1044/2018_AJA-17-0115

48. Berry J, Martin RL. You don't hear with your ears. *The Hearing Journal.* 2002;55:52-54.

49. Mealings K, Yeend I, Valderrama JT, et al. Discovering the unmet needs of people with difficulties understanding speech in noise and a normal or near-normal audiogram. *American Journal of Audiology.* 2020;29(3):329-355. doi:10.1044/2020_AJA-19-00093

50. Shub DE, Makashay MJ, Brungart DS. Predicting speech-in-noise deficits from the audiogram. *Ear and Hearing.* 2020;41(1):39-54. doi:10.1097/ AUD.0000000000000745

51. Henry JA, Trune DR, Robb MJA, Jastreboff PJ. *Tinnitus Retraining Therapy: Clinical Guidelines.* Plural Publishing, Inc.; 2007.

52. Henry JA, Zaugg TL, Myers PJ, Schechter MA. Using therapeutic sound with progressive audiologic tinnitus management. *Trends in Amplification.* 2008;12(3):188-209. doi:10.1177/1084713808321184

53. Jastreboff PJ. Optimal sound use in TRT—theory and practice. In: Hazell JWP, ed. *Proceedings of the Sixth International Tinnitus Seminar 1999.* The Tinnitus and Hyperacusis Centre; 1999:491-494.

54. Henry JA, Roberts LE, Caspary DM, Theodoroff SM, Salvi RJ. Underlying mechanisms of tinnitus: review and clinical implications. *Journal of the American Academy of Audiology.* 2014;25(1):5-22. doi:10.3766/jaaa.25.1.2

55. Jastreboff PJ. Phantom auditory perception (tinnitus): mechanisms of generation and perception. *Neuroscience Research.* 1990;8(4):221-54. doi:10.1016/0168-0102(90)90031-9

56. Kaltenbach JA, Zhang J, Zacharek MA. Neural correlates of tinnitus. In: Snow JB, ed. *Tinnitus: Theory and Management.* BC Decker; 2004:141-161.

57. Shore SE. Sensory nuclei in tinnitus. In: Snow JB, ed. *Tinnitus: .* BC Decker; 2004:125-139.

58. Kaltenbach JA, Godfrey DA, Neumann JB, McCaslin DL, Afman CE, Zhang J. Changes in spontaneous neural activity in the dorsal cochlear nucleus following exposure to intense sound: relation to threshold shift. *Hearing Research.* 1998;124(1-2):78-84. doi:10.1016/s0378-5955(98)00119-1

59. Heller MF, Bergman M. Tinnitus aurium in normally hearing persons. *Annals of Otology Rhinology and Laryngology.* 1953;62(1):73-83. doi:10.1177/000348945306200107

60. Henry JA, Reavis KM, Griest SE, et al. Tinnitus: an epidemiologic perspective. *Otolaryngology Clinics of North America*. 2020;53(4):481-499. doi:10.1016/j.otc.2020.03.002

61. Fagelson M. Tinnitus and traumatic memory. *Brain Science*. 2022;12(11)doi:10.3390/brainsci12111585

62. Kreuzer PM, Landgrebe M, Vielsmeier V, Kleinjung T, De Ridder D, Langguth B. Trauma-associated tinnitus. *Journal of Head Trauma Rehabilitation*. 2014;29(5):432-42. doi:10.1097/HTR.0b013e31829d3129

63. Carlson NR. *Physiology of Behavior*. Allyn and Bacon; 1991.

64. Hazell JWP. Support for a neurophysiological model of tinnitus. In: Reich GE, Vernon JA, eds. *Proceedings of the Fifth International Tinnitus Seminar*. American Tinnitus Association; 1996:51-57.

65. Rice CG. Annoyance due to low frequency hums. *BMJ*. 1994;308(6925):355-6. doi:10.1136/bmj.308.6925.355

66. Konorski J. *Conditioned Reflexes and Neuronal Organization*. Cambridge University Press; 1948.

67. Kehoe EJ, Macrae M. Classical conditioning. In: O'Donohue W, ed. *Learning and Behavioral Therapy*. Allyn & Bacon; 1998:36-58.

68. Grewal R, Spielmann PM, Jones SE, Hussain SS. Clinical efficacy of tinnitus retraining therapy and cognitive behavioural therapy in the treatment of subjective tinnitus: a systematic review. *Journal of Laryngology and Otology.* 2014;128(12):1028-33. doi:10.1017/S0022215114002849

69. Henry JA, Schechter MA, Zaugg TL, et al. Clinical trial to compare tinnitus masking and tinnitus retraining therapy. *Acta Oto-Laryngologica Supplementum.* 2006;(556):64-9. doi:10.1080/03655230600895556

70. Henry JA, Loovis C, Montero M, et al. Randomized clinical trial: group counseling based on tinnitus retraining therapy. *Journal of Rehabilitative Research and Development.* 2007;44(1):21-32. doi:10.1682/jrrd.2006.02.0018

71. Westin VZ, Schulin M, Hesser H, et al. Acceptance and Commitment Therapy versus Tinnitus Retraining Therapy in the treatment of tinnitus: a randomised controlled trial. *Behaviour Research and Therapy.* 2011;49(11):737-47. doi:10.1016/j.brat.2011.08.001

72. Tyler RS, Noble W, Coelho CB, Ji H. Tinnitus retraining therapy: mixing point and total masking are equally effective. *Ear and Hearing.* 2012;33(5):588-94. doi:10.1097/AUD.0b013e31824f2a6e

73. Henry JA, Stewart BJ, Griest S, Kaelin C, Zaugg TL, Carlson K. Multisite randomized controlled trial to compare two methods of tinnitus intervention to two control conditions. *Ear and Hearing.* 2016;37(6):e346-e359. doi:10.1097/AUD.0000000000000330

74. Bauer CA, Berry JL, Brozoski TJ. The effect of tinnitus retraining therapy on chronic tinnitus: A controlled trial. *Laryngoscope Investigative Otolaryngology.* 2017;2(4):166-177. doi:10.1002/lio2.76

75. Scherer RW, Formby C. Effect of Tinnitus Retraining Therapy vs standard of care on tinnitus-related quality of life: A randomized clinical trial. *JAMA Otolaryngology Head and Neck Surgery.* 2019;145(7):597-608. doi:10.1001/jamaoto.2019.0821

76. Vernon JA. Relief of tinnitus by masking treatment. In: English GM, ed. *Otolaryngology.* Harper & Row; 1982:1-21.

77. Dobie RA. A review of randomized clinical trials in tinnitus. *Laryngoscope.* 1999;109(8):1202-11. doi:10.1097/00005537-199908000-00004

78. Kilic C, Curran HV, Noshirvani H, Marks IM, Basoglu M. Long-term effects of alprazolam on memory: a 3.5 year follow-up of agoraphobia/panic patients. *Psychology Medicine.* 1999;29(1):225-31. doi:10.1017/s003329179800734x

79. Margolis RH. Audiology information counseling—what do patients remember? *Audiology Today.* 2004;16(2):14-15.

80. Shapiro DE, Boggs SR, Melamed BG, Graham-Pole J. The effect of varied physician affect on recall, anxiety, and perceptions in women at risk for breast cancer: an analogue study. *Health Psychology.* 1992;11(1):61-6. doi:10.1037//0278-6133.11.1.61

81. Kessels RP. Patients' memory for medical information. *Journal of the Royal Society of Medicine.* 2003;96(5):219-22. doi:10.1177/014107680309600504

82. Henry JA, Schechter MA, Zaugg TL, et al. Outcomes of clinical trial: tinnitus masking versus tinnitus retraining therapy. *Journal of the American Academy of Audiology.* 2006;17(2):104-32. doi:10.3766/jaaa.17.2.4

83. Lutman ME, Brown EJ, Coles RR. Self-reported disability and handicap in the population in relation to pure-tone threshold, age, sex and type of hearing loss. *British Journal of Audiology.* 1987;21(1):45-58. doi:10.3109/03005368709077774

84. Horwitz RI, Horwitz SM. Adherence to treatment and health outcomes. *Archives of Internal Medicine.* 1993;153(16):1863-8.

85. Jastreboff PJ, Jastreboff MM. Tinnitus Retraining Therapy for patients with tinnitus and decreased sound tolerance. *Otolaryngologic Clinics of North America.* 2003;36(2):321-36. doi:10.1016/s0030-6665(02)00172-x

86. Tyler RS, ed. *Tinnitus Treatment: Clinical Protocols.* Thieme; 2005.

87. Henry JA. Optimizing Tinnitus Retraining Therapy success. *Tinnitus Today.* 2002;27:16-17.

88. Henry JA, Carlson KF, Theodoroff S, Folmer RL. Reevaluating the use of sound therapy for tinnitus management: Perspectives on relevant systematic reviews. *Journal of Speech Language and Hearing Research.* 2022;65(6):2327-2342. doi:10.1044/2022_JSLHR-21-00668

89. Fuller T, Cima R, Langguth B, Mazurek B, Vlaeyen JW, Hoare DJ. Cognitive Behavioural Therapy for tinnitus. *Cochrane Database Systematic Review.* 2020;1(1):CD012614. doi:10.1002/14651858.CD012614. pub2

90. Hobson J, Chisholm E, El Refaie A. Sound therapy (masking) in the management of tinnitus in adults. *Cochrane Database Systematic Review.* 2012;11(11):CD006371. doi:10.1002/14651858.CD006371. pub3

91. Hoare DJ, Edmondson-Jones M, Sereda M, Akeroyd MA, Hall D. Amplification with hearing aids for patients with tinnitus and co-existing hearing loss. *Cochrane Database Systematic Review.* 2014;(1):CD010151. doi:10.1002/14651858.CD010151. pub2

92. Langguth B, Kleinjung T, Schlee W, Vanneste S, De Ridder D. Tinnitus guidelines and their evidence base. *Journal of Clinical Medicine.* 2023;12(9) doi:10.3390/jcm12093087

93. Schechter MA, Henry JA. Assessment and treatment of tinnitus patients using a "masking approach". *Journal of the American Academy of Audiology.* 2002;13(10):545-58.

94. Phillips JS, McFerran D. Tinnitus Retraining Therapy (TRT) for tinnitus. *Cochrane Database Systematic Review.* 2010;2010(3):CD007330. doi:10.1002/14651858.CD007330.pub2

95. Chandrasekhar SS, Tsai Do BS, Schwartz SR, et al. Clinical practice guideline: Sudden hearing loss (update). *Otolaryngology Head and Neck Surgery.* 2019;161(1_suppl):S1-S45. doi:10.1177/0194599819859885

96. Sismanis A. Pulsatile tinnitus. *Otolaryngologic Clinics of North America.* 2003;36(2):389-402, viii. doi:10.1016/s0030-6665(02)00169-x

97. Sismanis A. Evaluation and management of pulsatile tinnitus. In: Hughes GB, Pensak ML, eds. *Clinical Otology.* Thieme; 2007:476-486.

98. Fulbright ANC, Le Prell CG, Griffiths SK, Lobarinas E. Effects of recreational noise on threshold and suprathreshold measures of auditory function. *Seminars in Hearing.* 2017;38(4):298-318. doi:10.1055/s-0037-1606325

99. Axelsson A, Prasher D. Tinnitus induced by occupational and leisure noise. *Noise and Health.* 2000;2(8):47-54.

100. Salvi R, Auerbach BD, Lau C, et al. Functional neuro-anatomy of salicylate- and noise-induced tinnitus and hyperacusis. *Current Topics in Behavioral Neuroscience.* 2021;51:133-160. doi:10.1007/7854_2020_156

101. Dille MF, Konrad-Martin D, Gallun F, et al. Tinnitus onset rates from chemotherapeutic agents and ototoxic antibiotics: results of a large prospective study. *Journal of the American Academy of Audiology.* 2010;21(6):409-17. doi:10.3766/jaaa.21.6.6

102. DiSogra RM. Common aminoglycosides and platinum-based ototoxic drugs: Cochlear/vestibular side effects and incidence. *Seminars in Hearing.* 2019;40(2):104-107. doi:10.1055/s-0039-1684040

103. Altissimi G, Colizza A, Cianfrone G, et al. Drugs inducing hearing loss, tinnitus, dizziness and vertigo: an updated guide. *European Review for Medical and Pharmacological Sciences.* 2020;24(15):7946-7952. doi:10.26355/eurrev_202008_22477

104. Korres G, Kitsos DK, Kaski D, et al. The prevalence of dizziness and vertigo in COVID-19 patients: A systematic review. *Brain Science.* 2022;12(7)doi:10.3390/brainsci12070948

105. Bisdorff A, Von Brevern M, Lempert T, Newman-Toker DE. Classification of vestibular symptoms: towards an international classification of vestibular disorders. *Journal of Vestibular Research.* 2009;19(1-2):1-13. doi:10.3233/VES-2009-0343

106. Alsarhan H. Identification of early-stage Meniere's disease as a cause of unilateral tinnitus. *J Otol.* 2021;16(2):85-88. doi:10.1016/j.joto.2020.11.001

107. Mozaffari K, Zhang AB, Wilson B, et al. Evaluation of superior semicircular canal dehiscence anatomical location and clinical outcomes: A single institution's experience. *World Neurosurgery.* 2022;167:e865-e870. doi:10.1016/j.wneu.2022.08.090

108. Salem N, Galal A, Piras G, et al. Management of vestibular schwannoma with normal hearing. *Audiology and Neurotology.* 2023;28(1):12-21. doi:10.1159/000524925

109. Durai M, Searchfield G. Anxiety and depression, personality traits relevant to tinnitus: A scoping review. *International Journal of Audiology.* 2016;55(11):605-15. doi:10.1080/14992027.2016.1198966

110. Bartels H, Middel BL, van der Laan BF, Staal MJ, Albers FW. The additive effect of co-occurring anxiety and depression on health status, quality of life and coping strategies in help-seeking tinnitus sufferers. *Ear and Hearing.* 2008;29(6):947-56. doi:10.1097/AUD.0b013e3181888f83

111. Strumila R, Lengvenyte A, Vainutiene V, Lesinskas E. The role of questioning environment, personality traits, depressive and anxiety symptoms in tinnitus severity perception. *Psychiatry Quarterly.* 2017;88(4):865-877. doi:10.1007/s11126-017-9502-2

112. Salazar JW, Meisel K, Smith ER, Quiggle A, McCoy DB, Amans MR. Depression in patients with tinnitus: A systematic review. *Otolaryngology Head and Neck Surgery*. 2019;161(1):28-35. doi:10.1177/0194599819835178

113. Spitzer RL, Kroenke K, Williams JB, Lowe B. A brief measure for assessing generalized anxiety disorder: the GAD-7. *Archives of Internal Medicine*. 2006;166(10):1092-7. doi:10.1001/archinte.166.10.1092

114. Rutter LA, Brown TA. Psychometric properties of the Generalized Anxiety Disorder Scale-7 (GAD-7) in outpatients with anxiety and mood disorders. *Journal of Psychopathological Behavioral Assessment*. 2017;39(1):140-146. doi:10.1007/s10862-016-9571-9

115. Plummer F, Manea L, Trepel D, McMillan D. Screening for anxiety disorders with the GAD-7 and GAD-2: a systematic review and diagnostic meta-analysis. *General Hospital Psychiatry*. 2016;39:24-31. doi:10.1016/j.genhosppsych.2015.11.005

116. Kroenke K, Spitzer RL, Williams JB. The PHQ-9: validity of a brief depression severity measure. *Journal of General Internal Medicine*. 2001;16(9):606-13. doi:10.1046/j.1525-1497.2001.016009606.x

117. Martin A, Rief W, Klaiberg A, Braehler E. Validity of the Brief Patient Health Questionnaire Mood Scale (PHQ-9) in the general population. *General Hospital Psychiatry*. 2006;28(1):71-7. doi:10.1016/j.genhosppsych.2005.07.003

118. Erlandsson S. Psychological profiles of tinnitus patients. In: Tyler RS, ed. *Tinnitus Handbook*. Singular; 2000:25-57.

119. Bastien CH, Vallieres A, Morin CM. Validation of the Insomnia Severity Index as an outcome measure for insomnia research. *Sleep Medicine*. 2001;2(4):297-307. doi:10.1016/s1389-9457(00)00065-4

120. Morin CM, Belleville G, Belanger L, Ivers H. The Insomnia Severity Index: psychometric indicators to detect insomnia cases and evaluate treatment response. *Sleep*. 2011;34(5):601-8. doi:10.1093/sleep/34.5.601

121. Lan T, Cao Z, Zhao F, Perham N. The association between effectiveness of tinnitus intervention and cognitive function-a systematic review. *Frontiers in Psychology*. 2020;11:553449. doi:10.3389/fpsyg.2020.553449

122. Clarke NA, Henshaw H, Akeroyd MA, Adams B, Hoare DJ. Associations between subjective tinnitus and cognitive performance: systematic review and meta-analyses. *Trends in Hearing*. 2020;24:2331216520918416. doi:10.1177/2331216520918416

123. Sherlock LP, Brungart DS. Functional impact of bothersome tinnitus on cognitive test performance. *International Journal of Audiology*. 2021;60(12):1000-1008. doi:10.1080/14992027.2021.1909760

124. Brueggemann P, Neff PKA, Meyer M, Riemer N, Rose M, Mazurek B. On the relationship between tinnitus distress, cognitive performance and aging. *Progress in Brain Research.* 2021;262:263-285. doi:10.1016/bs.pbr.2021.01.028

125. Nagaratnam JM, Sharmin S, Diker A, Lim WK, Maier AB. Trajectories of Mini-Mental State Examination scores over the lifespan in general populations: a systematic review and meta-regression analysis. *Clinical Gerontology.* 2022;45(3):467-476. doi:10.1080/07317115.2020.1756021

126. Henry JA. Distinguishing between hearing loss, tinnitus, and hyperacusis: A recommended tinnitus-evaluation protocol for audiologists. *Tinnitus Today.* 2020;45(1):22-27.

127. Kim DK, Park SN, Kim HM, et al. Prevalence and significance of high-frequency hearing loss in subjectively normal-hearing patients with tinnitus. *Annals of Otology Rhinolology and Laryngology.* 2011;120(8):523-8. doi:10.1177/000348941112000806

128. Henry JA, Piskosz M, Norena A, Fournier P. Audiologists and tinnitus. *American Journal of Audiology.* 2019;28(4):1059-1064. doi:10.1044/2019_AJA-19-0070

129. Husain FT, Gander PE, Jansen JN, Shen S. Expectations for tinnitus teatment and outcomes: a survey study of audiologists and patients. *Journal of the American Academy of Audiology.* 2018;29(4):313-336. doi:10.3766/jaaa.16154

130. Henry JA, Sonstroem A, Smith B, Grush L. Survey of audiology graduate programs: training students in tinnitus management. *American Journal of Audiology.* 2021;30(1):22-27. doi:10.1044/2020_AJA-20-00140

131. Jafari Z, Baguley D, Kolb BE, Mohajerani MH. A systematic review and meta-analysis of extended high-frequency hearing thresholds in tinnitus with a normal audiogram. *Ear and Hearing.* 2022;43(6):1643-1652. doi:10.1097/AUD.0000000000001229

132. Peng F, Xiang Y, Xu H, Yin Q, Li J, Zou Y. Systematic review and meta-analysis of extended high-frequency audiometry in tinnitus patients. *Annals of Palliative Medicine.* 2021;10(12):12129-12139. doi:10.21037/apm-21-3060

133. Jastreboff MM, Jastreboff PJ. Decreased sound tolerance and Tinnitus Retraining Therapy (TRT). *Australian and New Zealand Journal of Audiology.* 2002;24:74-81.

134. Formby C, Gold SL. Modification of loudness discomfort level: evidence for adaptive chronic auditory gain and its clinical relevance. *Seminars in Hearing.* 2002;23:21-35.

Index

inner versus outer hair cells 88, 90

loss of inner hair cells 90

loss of outer hair cells 89, 90

organ of Corti 86, 88, 89

otoacoustic emissions 91

middle ear 84

eardrum 84, 86, 204

ossicles 86, 204

neural networks 93, 96

nuclei (brain centers) 85

outer ear 84

ear canal 84, 86

tonotopic organization 92

two major divisions 83

auditory nervous system 83

the ear 83

Heller and Bergman experiment 94, 130

importance of 95

results 94

hypnosis 105

stochastic resonance 74, 234
stress 48, 110, 113
  consequences of 108
  management 132
  stressful relationships 147
  tinnitus and 108
superior canal dehiscence 199

T

threshold of audibility 74
tinnitus
  activities affected by 54, 151
  annoyance 153, 154
  asymmetric 42
  awareness of 153, 182
  bad days 48, 147
  bothersome versus not bothersome 104
  cause, theoretical
    discordant damage or dysfunction of hair cells 91, 130
  constant 43, 119
  cure
    definition 4
    lack of 12, 60, 122, 168
  definition 43, 173
  educational counseling 189
  effects of 11, 12, 113, 182
  emotional reactions 111, 153, 154
  fears associated with 116
  fluctuating 43, 169
  functional effects 53
  generator 122
  impact 155
  intermittent 43, 119
  loudness 57, 140, 154
    decrease in the perception of 168
    increasing 148
  masking 71, 137
  masking method of treatment 185, 189
  matching 47
  neural signal 135
    blocking of 111, 126, 174
    important versus unimportant 101
    making detection more difficult 136
    reducing the strength of 129, 135, 136
    relative strength of 135
  new-onset 122
  no-problem 111
  objective 196
  perceived as threatening 102
  persistent 34, 45, 197
  primary 34, 195
  problem 110, 111, 115, 150, 157
  prolonged worsening 217
  pulsatile 197
  quality. *See* tinnitus:spectral characteristics
  reactions 58
  recent-onset 45, 197
  reclassification to a neutral signal 130, 133
  secondary 195
  sensation of 11
  side effect of normal compensation 130
  sleep deprivation due to 54
  spectral characteristics 72
    changing 75
  spiking 49, 169
  sudden-onset 7, 197
  suppression 71
    complete 72, 137

Dr. Henry spent most of his 35-year career as an independent researcher testing and developing methods of clinical management for tinnitus. He is one of the world's leading experts in how to evaluate and treat tinnitus. His efforts are now focused on writing books about tinnitus, hyperacusis, and hearing loss—all under the heading of Ears Gone Wrong. These books are intended for the general public to be easily understood with practical information for addressing these auditory challenges.

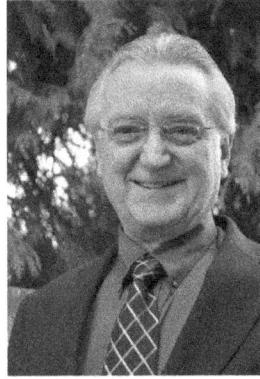

www.earsgonewrong.org

Sign up today for my free monthly newsletter and receive instant access to my upcoming books, posts, and information about tinnitus.

To subscribe, please scan the QR Code below, or go to http://earsgonewrong.org

Password for QR Code: earsgonewrong

Scan me!

www.ingramcontent.com/pod-product-compliance
Lightning Source LLC
Chambersburg PA
CBHW032051020426
42335CB00011B/283